CW01512416

—— THE ESSENCE OF ——

BIPOLAR DISORDER

THE ESSENCE OF

BIPOLAR DISORDER

Based on Progress in Neuroscience and Genetics

William J. Walsh, PhD

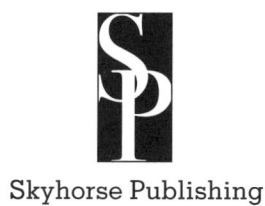

Skyhorse Publishing

Skyhorse Publishing books may be purchased in bulk at special discounts for sales promotion, corporate gifts, fund-raising, or educational purposes. Special editions can also be created to specifications. For details, contact the Special Sales Department, Skyhorse Publishing, 307 West 36th Street, 11th Floor, New York, NY 10018 or info@skyhorsepublishing.com.

Skyhorse® and Skyhorse Publishing® are registered trademarks of Skyhorse Publishing, Inc.®, a Delaware corporation.

Visit our website at www.skyhorsepublishing.com.
Please follow our publisher Tony Lyons on Instagram @tonylyonsisuncertain

10 9 8 7 6 5 4 3 2 1

Library of Congress Cataloging-in-Publication Data is available on file.

Cover theme by Freepik
Cover design by Tim Rohlwing and Katherine Kubik

Print ISBN: 978-1-5107-8597-7
Ebook ISBN: 978-1-5107-8598-4

Printed in the United States of America

Dedication

This book is dedicated to Dr. Robert A. de Vito, a brilliant psychiatrist and my best friend. We met when he was Chairman of the Department of Psychiatry at Loyola Stritch School of Medicine and Chief of Psychiatry at Loyola University Medical Center, and I joined his national team studying serial killers. Over the next 20 years, I learned he was a secret Good Samaritan who regularly ventured into dangerous Chicago neighborhoods to provide free services to the mentally ill. I often hear from psychiatrists he trained and former patients who speak of his great intellect and dedication to help others. In 2018, he was named a Distinguished Fellow by the American Psychiatric Association (APA's highest honor). Our friendship led to more than 800 weekly lunches at Italian restaurants where we had a jolly good time, but we also discussed mental illness and exciting new brain research. One day we shared our unhappiness at psychiatry's inability to understand bipolar disorder and the limited effectiveness of clinical treatments. Within 30 minutes we developed a plan in which I would explore recent neuroscience research, seeking answers to the many mysteries surrounding the condition. Although he had retired to care for his ailing wife, Dr. Bob actively reviewed the early findings and provided helpful editing when I started writing this book. His life serves as a model for physicians who are dedicated to making the world a better place.

Disclaimer

The clinical therapies described in this book require supervision by an experienced medical professional. Bipolar disorder is a complex condition, and improper treatments can have a powerful effect on brain functioning that can cause harm. Readers must not attempt self-treatment based on information in this book.

The case histories in this book provide examples of medical challenges, treatment approaches, and experiences of real patients. Names and certain other information have been changed to assure patient confidentiality. Individual patient outcomes are intended to illustrate clinical interventions and should not be regarded as evidence of treatment effectiveness.

The book's use of the term "mental illness" and descriptions of individual symptoms and behaviors is descriptive only, and no disrespect is intended to the persons challenged by bipolar disorder. The principal objective of this volume is to provide information that may help researchers and clinicians improve the quality of life of individuals challenged by this illness.

Acknowledgments

After 35 years researching mental disorders and trying to help 30,000 patients, I wrote *Nutrient Power*, a book summarizing recent clinical advances and promising new treatments for behavior disorders, ADHD, autism, depression, schizophrenia, and Alzheimer's disease. However, the book did not include a chapter on bipolar disorder despite having worked with hundreds of patients with the diagnosis. I believed there simply was not enough known about this very mysterious mental illness to write a meaningful chapter that might benefit clinicians and their patients. Basic bipolar unknowns included the cause, genetic predispositions, reasons for delayed onset after many years of relative normality, and mechanisms that could explain switching between mania and depression. About 10 years ago, I became very excited about major progress in brain science and decided to search for bipolar insights from recent published research. Dr. Robert de Vito spent hundreds of hours patiently answering questions about complex neuroscience and treatment alternatives. He would have been co-author of this book except for declining health and an early death.

My experience in mental illness began when the renowned Dr. Carl Pfeiffer of Princeton, New Jersey, became interested in my biochemical studies of violent criminals. We began a friendship of many years that included collaborative treatment of hundreds of patients diagnosed with schizophrenia or behavior disorders. I enjoyed working with many dedicated and capable clinicians, especially Drs. Robert Thomas, Laura Glab, Albert Mensah, Judy Bowman, and Malcolm Sickels, who taught important lessons about patient care and clinical protocols. It was both educational and inspiring working with hundreds of brave patients challenged by bipolar disorder. I am very appreciative of the efforts of board officers Jack Provenzale and Ed Tanzman as well as numerous board members who volunteered their time. Staff members Sue Hanegraaf and Dana Zingrone were the first to suggest this book and capably directed Walsh Research

Institute activities for years. I would be lost without Lisa Pecho and Deloris Janke who are now fulfilling this role. Katherine Kubik organized the manuscript, created illustrations, and provided important neuroscience information. Research interns Nicole Coates, Kendall Gaspari, Pujan Vyas, Khushali Vyas, and Isaac Noren assisted in the extensive search of available scientific literature. Thanks go to my talented editor, Teri Arranga, who also edited my earlier book *Nutrient Power.* Eva Edelman provided a helpful and detailed review of the manuscript. Professional illustrators Caroline O'Ryan and Tim Rohlwing designed most of the illustrations. Accountant Dipika Vyas has brought financial stability to our charity for several years. The Hilton Family Foundation provided financial support for schizophrenia research studies that led to mental health insights important to this investigation.

One morning in 1986, my wife, Barbara, suggested that I quit my comfortable job at Argonne National Laboratory to pursue my independent research into violent crime and mental disorders. Her willingness to accept this financial risk while raising 5 children allowed me to devote the rest of my life to the study of mental illnesses. My life changed that morning; without her constant support and encouragement, my work and this book would not have been possible.

Contents

Foreword

This book describes a multiyear investigation that may have identified the cause of bipolar disorder and provides a detailed explanation for chronic cycling between mania and clinical depression. This effort was born out of frustration. By 2014, my colleagues and I had worked with more than 1,500 patients diagnosed with bipolar disorder and witnessed their severe mental pain and the burden on their families. Although most of our patients reported improvements, only a small percentage could achieve a truly satisfying recovery. A major barrier has been the inability of medical science to understand the basic causes and mechanisms of this unique mental illness. For more than a century, clinical advances have been hampered by the many unknowns that shroud bipolar disorder. It is difficult to fight an enemy if you don't know who or what it is.

My original plan was to spend six months exploring recent advances in neuroscience searching for bipolar disorder insights. In a very short time, I found thousands of researchers scattered throughout the world studying the complex mechanisms of the human brain and learned that great progress had been achieved. My investigation grew into a fascinating multiyear exploration of exciting new findings in genetics, epigenetics, glial cells, methylation, ion channels, DNA damage, and other fields that are revolutionizing our understanding of the brain. Eventually, I was able to develop promising explanations for many mysteries associated with bipolar disorder. A novel analysis of recent genomic findings identified specific DNA variants associated with bipolar disorder predisposition. Progressive DNA damage considerations led to the cause of bipolar disorder's late onset and a likely mechanism for mania/depression switching. This book presents a new theory that attempts to explain the very essence of bipolar disorder. If this model is correct, it could lead to vastly improved therapies and perhaps prevention of this very cruel disorder.

To a large degree, this book is based on research by others. I salute the world's dedicated neuroscientists who continue the ironic task of using their brains to discover how brains work.

Exploring the Mysteries of Bipolar Disorder

In 1939, Winston Churchill described Russia as "a riddle wrapped in a mystery inside an enigma." Today these words could be used to describe bipolar disorder. Also known as manic depression, this illness has existed in society for thousands of years but has only been actively researched since the early 1900s. Despite a century of intensive research, the basic causes and mechanisms have remained elusive. More than seventy million[1] are challenged by this disorder that continues to be a leading cause of suicide, unemployment, and loss of human potential. Bipolar disorder usually begins in the late teens or early adulthood with an unexpected onset of mania that typically worsens until the condition mysteriously switches into an episode of clinical depression. Bipolar disorder is a unique mental illness characterized by alternating periods of mania and depression that can have a devastating effect on both career and family life. The suicide rate for this illness is higher than the rates for schizophrenia, clinical depression, and anxiety disorders. Psychiatric medications have helped many, but their benefits are usually partial in nature and often involve unpleasant side effects. Counseling often improves the quality of life but usually falls well short of recovery. After more than a century of research, fundamental unknowns continue to hinder the development of truly effective therapies:

- What is the essential cause of bipolar disorder?
- What changes in the brain can explain the massive impairment in functioning?

- Why doesn't the illness go away after onset despite a century of aggressive treatments?
- Why does prolonged mania descend into clinical depression?
- Why does mania tend to return after weeks or months of depression?
- What can explain the chronic switching between mania and depression that can persist for a lifetime?

In this investigation, I explored recent neuroscience advances in an attempt to resolve some of these unknowns. Although most bipolar research is aimed at the development of improved drug medications, scientists are making revolutionary advances in understanding the extraordinary complexity of the brain. I was surprised to learn there are more than 250,000 neuroscientists throughout the world and found impressive research in unexpected places like Iceland, Albania, and Turkey. The past 20 years have seen an exponential increase in brain research with hundreds of new studies published each month. It took more than a year to become familiar with the major advances in neuroscience since the year 2000. Due to the immense amount of new neuroscience information, my plan to devote six months seeking bipolar insights developed into an exciting multiyear project. Especially helpful were many excellent survey articles in peer-reviewed journals that summarized progress in specific areas of brain research. It was a constant challenge to keep abreast of important new research every month. Scientific conferences were great opportunities to follow new research and engage in discussions with leaders in the field. My favorite has been the annual gathering of the Society for Neuroscience that typically attracts more than 20,000 attendees from about 80 countries. The National Institute of Mental Health (NIMH) has been an excellent source of detailed information regarding bipolar disorder. I also learned new information whenever I attended annual meetings of the American Psychiatric Association. Progress in brain science is advancing so rapidly that some neuroscience books published after 2015 are already obsolete.

This book presents a history of this investigation. The first chapters summarize the history and present clinical status of bipolar disorder and share lessons learned in working with 1,500 patients diagnosed with the condition. More than a year was devoted to identification of factors with high significance in bipolar disorder; factors included epi-genetics, ion channels, glial cells, DNA nourishment of cell types, DNA damage, DNA repair, and breakthroughs in genetic research. An early focus was bipolar disorder's typical severe oxidative over-load associated with damaging free radicals that assault DNA. An analysis concluded that bipolar disorder is a late-onset DNA-damage illness involving strong genetic predispositions with creation of newly mutated genes with advancing age. A novel analysis of recent genomic advances identified the primary predisposing factors that cause bipo-lar disorder. This led to detailed explanations for mania onset, the switch to temporary depression, and permanent tendency for mania/depression cycling. This book does not describe the many blind alleys and unsuccessful studies that prolonged this investigation. The final chapters present a comprehensive novel theory of bipolar disorder that attempts to describe the essence of bipolar disorder.

CHAPTER 1

Bipolar Disorder –
A Capsule Summary

Historical Perspective

Bipolar disorder, also known as manic depression, is a mental disorder distinguished by alternating periods of excitability (mania) and depression.[1] References to depression are found in our earliest recorded history, and mania was described by the ancient Greeks. The first physician to identify the unique symptoms of bipolar disorder was Aretaeus in the second century A.D.[2] However, the condition was not recognized as a major mental disorder until 1854 when French psychiatrist Jean-Pierre Falret[3] reported a disorder he called "la folie circulaire," described as "a continuous cycle of depression, mania and free intervals of varying length." A major advance in the understanding of bipolar disorder is credited to the German psychiatrist Emil Kraepelin, who published the distinction between manic depressive illness and schizophrenia in 1919.[4] After many years, "bipolar disorder" has replaced the expression "manic depression" to avoid connotations with the word "maniac." Until 1950, most psychiatrists believed the illness resulted from flawed life experiences. Freud,[5] Adler,[6] Jung,[7] and others developed talk therapies and counseling techniques that focused on traumatic events or poor environments that were considered the cause of the disorder. These psychodynamic approaches became standard throughout the world of psychiatry for several decades. However, disappointing outcomes frequently led to lobotomy, electroshock therapy (also known as electroconvulsive therapy or ECT), and other highly-invasive therapies in a somewhat desperate attempt to help severely ill patients.

The Biochemical Revolution and Psychiatric Drugs: Research
advances during the 1950s and 1960s brought dramatic improvements in the basic understanding of mental illnesses. For example,
adoption[8] and twin studies[9,10] proved that the greatest predictor of
mental illness was not life experiences but rather a family history of
the same disorder. By the late 1960s, most scientific and medical
experts agreed that the essence of bipolar disorder and other mental
illnesses involved genetic chemical imbalances or other impairments
that alter neurotransmissions.[11,12] Within a few years, mainstream psychiatry changed its primary focus from life experiences to neurotransmitters (NTs), receptors, and the molecular biology of the brain.

    This was a difficult time for psychiatrists since much of what they
learned in medical school had become irrelevant. Since severely ill
patients were in desperate need of immediate improvement, prac-
titioners turned to psychiatric medications, which were the only
established therapies at that time for altering neurotransmitter activity.[13] Initial bipolar drug treatments focused on lithium (Li), anticonvulsants, and other medications aimed at coping with mania. Within
a few years, dopamine-lowering drugs such as Thorazine, Prolixin,
and Mellaril became treatments of choice for schizophrenia. Since
those early days, dozens of new psychiatric medications have been
developed, including antidepressants, benzodiazepines, and 2nd
generation antipsychotics (also called atypical antipsychotics). This
has evolved into a massive pharmaceutical industry with annual
sales of 20 billion dollars by 2025, with numerous pharmaceutical
companies and universities in a competitive race to develop the next
billion-dollar drug.[14,15]

    Medication therapies have helped millions of diagnosed bipolar
patients, but benefits are usually partial in nature with a high incidence of unpleasant side effects. Due to biochemical individuality,
drug therapy is often more art than science and involves a considerable amount of trial and error. A fundamental limitation is that most
psychiatric drugs are foreign molecules that result in an abnormal
condition, rather than producing normalcy in the brain. Most persons
with a bipolar diagnosis endure a disappointing quality of life despite
their doctor's dedicated attempts to help them.[16] There is universal
agreement in psychiatry that improved bipolar treatments are desper-
ately needed. The lion's share of today's research funds is aimed at

development of more effective drugs, with a lesser amount directed at the fundamental causes and mechanisms of bipolar disorder.

Bipolar Disorder – A Difficult Diagnosis

Bipolar disorder is a mental health condition characterized by extreme mood swings that fluctuate between emotional highs and depressive lows.[17] The median age at onset is 25 years. The illness often begins with some degree of mania, defined as a period of abnormally and persistently elevated, expansive, or irritable mood, coupled with increased goal-directed activity or energy and lasting at least one week.[18] Most manic episodes last weeks or months before being replaced by depression that may last many months. For some, the transitions can be quite sudden, while others may experience a period of normalcy before the next episode. In the absence of effective treatment, patients may cycle between mania and depression for the rest of their lives, plagued by extreme changes in mood, energy, concentration, and ability to perform basic tasks.

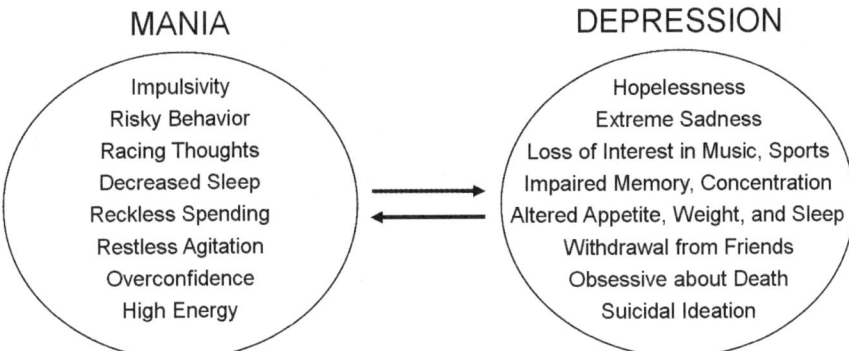

Due to genetic and epigenetic complexities, bipolar disorder has very different impacts for different individuals. If you went to a party attended by 100 people with a bipolar diagnosis, you might find it difficult to believe they shared the same illness. Bipolar disorder is a very democratic illness that can afflict anyone regardless of race, gender, intelligence level, financial status, physical health, or personality. According to the 2022 updated DSM-5-TR diagnostic manual for psychiatrists (*Diagnostic and Statistical Manual of Mental Disorders*, Fifth Edition, Text Revision), there are three primary types of bipolar disorder:

- *Bipolar 1 disorder*: This diagnosis involves recurring manic episodes that last at least one week, followed by major depressive periods of at least two weeks. The manic period represents a striking change from the person's usual behavior, which may include sleep problems, disorganized thinking, rapid speech, risky behavior, and spending sprees. Mania often becomes increasingly severe and may include hallucinations and delusional thoughts.[19] The transition to the depression phase may be sudden or gradual and is characterized by intense sadness or despair and loss of interest in previously enjoyable activities. During this period, a person may isolate themselves from others, be unable to work, and have persistent thoughts of suicide. Without successful treatment, the depression phase typically is replaced by return of mania and a lifetime of chronic cycling between mania and depression.
- *Bipolar 2 disorder*: This condition involves chronic cycling between depression and hypomania, a milder version of mania characterized by inflated self-esteem or grandiosity, decreased need for sleep, racing thoughts, hyperactivity, and a tendency for high-risk behaviors. A significant percentage of bipolar 2 disorder patients enjoy the hypomania phase and report heightened creativity, work productivity, and energy during this period. However, the euphoria and impulsivity often lead to high-risk and unwise behavior. I recall a capable and intelligent patient who bought two $100,000 boats on the same day, despite limited funds. Family and friends may be frightened by personality changes, nonstop talking, hypersexuality, irrational beliefs, or lack of sleep. The depression experienced in bipolar 2 is usually the most dangerous aspect of the condition, often involving extraordinary sadness, lack of pleasure in most activities, isolation from others, inability to work, despair, and suicidal ideation.
- *Cyclothymic disorder*: This condition involves chronic shifts between mild hypomanic and low-grade depressive symptoms that last at least 2 years but do not meet criteria for a major depressive, manic, or hypomanic episode. The symptoms mirror those of bipolar 2, though on a

smaller scale and usually are not incapacitating. However, the illness involves clinically significant distress or impaired social, occupational, or other important areas of functioning. Cyclothymic individuals typically can carry out their daily activities and have greatly reduced suicide risk compared to other bipolar individuals. They may benefit from counseling and rarely are treated with psychiatric drugs. This diagnosis is associated with a high risk for substance abuse.

Other Bipolar Disorder Descriptors: The term mixed states refers to bipolar 1, bipolar 2, or cyclothymia disorder in which symptoms of mania and depression occur either simultaneously or in very short succession. Since the 1980s, I evaluated hundreds of patients diagnosed with bipolar disorder who reported distinct mood swings between high anxiety and severe depression that might occur several times the same week. Interestingly, we also observed similar extreme mood swings in hundreds of patients who had no evidence of bipolar disorder. The two populations shared a high incidence of extreme oxidative overload, inflammation, and a metal metabolism disorder, usually involving zinc depletion. This has led me to suspect that the mixed states diagnosis used in bipolar patients may represent a con-comitant condition and not a variation of bipolar disorder.

Many of our clinical patients presented with a diagnosis of "bipolar disorder with rapid cycling" that refers to the presence of at least 4 episodes in the last twelve months that meet the criteria for a manic, hypomanic, or major depressive episode. In our experience, most of the rapid-cycle patients reported manic-depressive switches every few days or weeks with symptoms and biochemical imbalances that resembled mixed states patients.

Over the past two decades, an increasing number of patients have been diagnosed with a bipolar spectrum disorder, which is a condition that shares some features with bipolar phenotypes but fails to meet criteria for bipolar 1 disorder, bipolar 2 disorder, or cyclothymia. This includes many people who have never experienced a manic episode or patients who simply respond to lithium or other bipolar medica-tions. I arbitrarily excluded patients diagnosed with mixed states, rapid cycling, or a spectrum disorder from my investigation to concentrate on the mechanisms and neuroscience of classic bipolar disorder.

The accuracy of bipolar disorder diagnoses is far from perfect despite the helpful definitions in DSM-5. For example, hundreds of our patients diagnosed with bipolar disorder have never experienced a manic episode, and their diagnosis is speculative. We have met many patients with nearly identical symptoms in which one was diagnosed with bipolar disorder and the other with schizophrenia. However, the 2022 revision of the DSM-5 has begun to cope with this problem. Although the median age of onset is 25 years, thousands of very young children and adolescents now receive a bipolar diagnosis and are treated with powerful 2nd generation antipsychotic drugs despite little or no evidence of a manic episode. It is difficult to have confidence in a diagnosis based on a prediction of mental deterioration in the distant future. In addition, there are thousands with a true bipolar disorder who have never been diagnosed and need medical attention.

Bipolar Disorder Treatments

More than two dozen medications are now available for mainstream treatment of bipolar disorder. Occasional patients do quite well on a single drug, but most patients are prescribed two or more simultaneously.[20] I once met a bipolar patient who was taking eleven separate medications daily. About one-fifth of all bipolar patients receive four or more psychotropic medications, although the safety and efficacy of these combinations have never been tested in systematic studies.[21,22] Most randomized studies of bipolar drug combinations have focused on efficacy of a single mood stabilizer with a specific atypical antipsychotic.

These therapeutics originally were referred to as psychiatric drugs, which later were termed as medications, and then most recently are called biologics (perhaps for marketing reasons). Medication selection may be based on a patient's symptoms, medical history, and the practitioner's experience with specific drugs. It is very difficult to predict a patient's response to any medication or medication combination, and trial and error are frequently necessary. The primary types of bipolar medications are the following:

- *Mood stabilizers*: Nearly all bipolar patients are treated with a medication aimed at controlling manic or hypomanic episodes. Examples of mood stabilizers include lithium, Depakote, Tegretol, and Lamictal. Several of these drugs are also mainstream treatments for epilepsy. Note that brand names are used for medications (rather than generic names) since this book is written for both professional and informed lay audiences.

- *Antipsychotics*: Over the past 10 years, schizophrenia drugs called atypical antipsychotics have been increasingly prescribed for bipolar disorder. Originally used for severe mania that involved psychosis, they are now commonly prescribed for non-psychotic bipolar patients to provide sedation and other beneficial features of these drugs. Examples include Zyprexa, Risperdal, Seroquel, Abilify, Geodon, Latuda, and Saphris. These medications typically are used in combination with a mood stabilizer.
- *Antidepressants*: Antidepressants are often prescribed to help manage the depression phase of bipolar disorder. However, they must be used carefully to avoid triggering a manic episode and are usually prescribed together with a mood stabilizer.
- *Anti-anxiety medications*: Xanax, Klonopin, Valium, or other benzodiazepines may help with anxiety or sleep by increasing neurotransmission of the inhibitory NT gamma-aminobutyric acid (GABA) in the brain. However, these medications have a high addiction profile and are usually provided on a short-term basis.

Treatment of bipolar disorder is very challenging since the condition involves two quite opposite mental disorders (mania and depression) in the same person. The transitions between mania and depression can be very rapid, and each phase requires a different treatment approach. Even the most-nimble practitioner finds it challenging to quickly change treatment protocols during bipolar cycling. Recently there has been a movement to develop single drugs that are effective for both mania and depression phases of the disorder. For example, the new medication Vraylar mediates both mania and depression by enhancing activities at dopamine D_2 and serotonin 1A receptors, while repressing activity at serotonin 2A receptors. Aggressive medication therapies are used during acute bipolar episodes that may involve dangerous behavior and suicide risk. Hospitalization is often necessary if a patient presents a high risk of harm to self or others, and this can also be an ideal setting for medication trials that could possibly make things worse. After stabilization, medicated patients may benefit from a structured environment, counseling, and psychotherapy, but the support of family and friends may be even more important. Unfortunately, complete recoveries are relatively rare, and bipolar disorder typically results in a reduced quality of life that persists until the end of life.[23]

The Onset of Bipolar Disorder

Warning signs of mental dysfunction are often present before bipolar onset, but the disorder can also appear quite suddenly after years of normality. The average age of bipolar onset is 25 years, which usually begins with a serious episode of mania or hypomania. However, the disorder may develop in the teen years and in rare cases may affect young children.[24] Researchers have determined that mania generally begins with neuronal hyperactivity in specific brain locations and NT systems.[25] There is general agreement that bipolar disorder onset involves a combination of genetic predisposition together with mental trauma, physical injury, or environmental insults. For most people, the illness does not go away after onset and represents a difficult challenge for the rest of their lives. This suggests that bipolar onset is a life-changing event that causes a permanent impairment in brain stability that involves chronic cycling between mania and depression.

Since bipolar onset often begins during a period of severe mental or physical trauma, decades of psychiatric talk therapies have explored the nature of this trauma in an attempt to reverse the enduring psychic harm to a patient. However, triggering events may not provide a reliable guide to effective treatment. A careless cigarette may start a raging forest fire, but finding the cigarette will not help the firefighters. Epigenetic science has discovered that emotional or physical trauma can produce permanent adverse changes in gene expression that may result in a chronic mental illness. Psychotherapy and counseling have helped countless patients cope with bipolar disorder, but treatments to correct abnormal behavior of key NT systems may be more effective and enduring by addressing the dominant causes of bipolar disorder.

Many people diagnosed with bipolar disorder attempt to prevent friends and colleagues from knowing about their illness. They may hold responsible jobs and perform well during hypomania and transition phases, but they might collapse when depression strikes and suffer in isolation. Many individuals with bipolar 2 disorder are able to hide their mental disorder from employers and co-workers for several years. For example, George, age 35, had a college degree and excellent performance ratings with several companies, but he also had a history of jumping from job to job. He first developed hypomania at age 23 and was able to maintain productivity for more than a year until he experienced severe depression. He then resigned from his position and was unemployed for months until the depression faded away. This sequence of events repeated many times over the next 12 years. His excellent job ratings and references brought employment, but he was unable to function after six to eighteen months on each job. He finally sought medical help after his wife divorced him.

Mania experienced in bipolar 1 disorder usually follows a worsening trajectory. In the absence of effective treatment, mania usually becomes increasingly severe and may involve psychosis and hospitalization. Patients diagnosed with bipolar 1 generally are unable to hide the illness from friends and employers due to the more obvious symptoms of severe mania, and most seek medical help soon after onset. Hundreds of these patients described the dramatic and disconcerting changes during their initial manic episode. One such patient, Jack, age 28, was enjoying his job in downtown Chicago, but he then started having racing thoughts and sleep problems. Anti-anxiety medications helped for a few weeks, but his condition gradually worsened. One day driving back from work, he heard a voice he thought came from the back seat. He raced to the nearest police station expecting to be attacked. After a search found nobody in his car, he continued home but again heard the voice. He thought his fun-loving friends were playing a practical joke, but a search of the car failed to find any evidence of tampering. Two days later, the alleged voice started coming from his TV at home, and he went to the emergency room. His eventual diagnosis was bipolar 1 disorder with psychotic features, and his life was never the same again.

While most patients with a bipolar diagnosis experience a lifetime of misery and disappointment after onset, history provides examples of high achievement despite the condition. Winston Churchill was a heroic figure who inspired Great Britain and the world during World War II. Despite severe bipolar disorder, he managed to publish 43 books during his sleepless mania episodes and famously complained of his "black dog" of depression. Other historic examples include Isaac Newton, Charles Darwin, and Vincent van Gogh. Many of today's celebrities have achieved stardom despite their bipolar condition, including Ted Turner, Mel Gibson, Mariah Carey, Catherine Zeta-Jones, and Jane Pauley. This leads to the conclusion that bipolar disorder does not impair the entire brain since impressive cognition, artistic skills, and business acumen are still possible.

Heritability and Bipolar Disorder

Bipolar disorders exhibit a very strong genetic component compared to most other mental illnesses.[8,9,10,26] For example, children with two bipolar parents have a 75% lifetime risk for the same diagnosis when compared to 38% for children of two schizophrenic parents. In another example, bipolar's 75% concordance for identical twins is roughly double that of clinical depression. Recent research suggests that depression and schizophrenia are broad terms that each include a variety of illnesses that exhibit different symptoms and misbehaving NTs.[25] This might explain reduced heritability compared to bipolar disorder that may be a more singular mental disorder. Early twin studies proved genetic inheritance was bipolar disorder's primary risk factor, and the remainder was attributed to environmental insults. However, recent studies suggest that epigenetic variations in gene expression also contribute to bipolar disorder risk.[27,28] In any case, bipolar disorder runs very strongly in families and involves an unusually strong genetic component. Surprisingly, the first 30 years of genetic studies failed to find a single gene associated with the illness. Chapter 8 describes major advances in genomic research that have since identified dozens of low-effect gene variants that predispose to bipolar disorder.

Bipolar Disorder – A Deadly Mental Illness

Published studies indicate that bipolar disorder carries the highest suicide risk of all major mental illnesses. Between 25% and 50% of all bipolar patients attempt suicide at least once, and there is a lifetime suicide incidence of 15%.[29,30,31] In comparison, the equivalent suicide risk for schizophrenia is about 5%. Major depressive disorder (MDD) carries a lifetime suicide risk of 7% for males and 1% for females. For many years, the suicide risk for bipolar 1 disorder was believed to be much higher than that for bipolar 2 disorder. However, recent careful studies indicate that lifetime suicide risk is approximately 15% for both bipolar phenotypes.

There are several theories as to why bipolar disorder carries this extraordinary tendency for self-destruction. Compared with persons diagnosed with schizophrenia, those with bipolar (a) may have clearer insights regarding the severe damage the illness has done to their quality of life, career, and family, and (b) may be more capable at carrying out the task of suicide. In addition, bipolar depressions are very different from other mood disorders and may intrinsically involve more psychic pain. It is also possible that a sudden descent into bipolar depression may be more difficult to endure than a gradual transition into severe depression. In my experience, many patients become despondent and hopeless during a depression relapse, and forget progress previously attained. I recall an intelligent professional woman who sent our clinical staff flowers in gratitude for "ending her nightmare of bipolar 2." She returned to the office three weeks later with her first relapse in years and complained that our treatment had never helped her. I took her into the reception area and showed her the flowers and her note of thanks. She had lost all memory of the previous great improvement. Many patients receive benzodiazepine medications as a sleep aid or for calming, and these drugs are notorious for erasing memories. Also, sadly, at the home of caring, supportive families, patients may mislead themselves thinking suicide would ease the burden of their loved ones. Perhaps the greatest suicide risk factor is the typical inability of medications and other mainstream therapies to provide a satisfactory quality of life.

The Lithium Saga

In the late 1940s, Australian psychiatrist John Cade accidentally discovered the calming effect of lithium in a hospital's unused kitchen he had converted into a primitive research laboratory.[32,33,34] During crude experiments, Cade injected urine from mania patients into guinea pigs that were family pets in his backyard. Upon observing that urine from manic patients was quite toxic to his pigs, he began research on urea and uric acid, which were known to have toxic properties. Frustrated by the low solubility of uric acid in water, he added lithium salts to achieve higher uric acid concentrations for his experiments.

In a total surprise, he discovered lithium had a major calming effect on the guinea pigs. Cade started treating mania patients with lithium salts and reported striking improvements. Realizing that lithium is present in tiny concentrations in humans, he theorized that mania was caused by lithium deficiency. Soon, several doctors in Australia and elsewhere began treating mania with lithium and confirmed the benefits observed by Cade. Unfortunately, some patients developed kidney or liver damage from lithium, and there were several fatalities. The Food and Drug Administration (FDA) eventually banned the use of lithium medications in the USA and characterized it as a quack remedy, and many doctors were punished for providing lithium to patients. For several years, interest in lithium therapies in America nearly disappeared, while other countries continued to study medical uses of lithium.

In the 1960s, published studies reported that the incidence of depression, suicide, and criminality was surprisingly low in areas around Amarillo, Texas. Researchers soon discovered unusually high lithium levels in Amarillo's water supply, and this sparked renewed USA interest in medical uses of lithium. By the early 1970s, there was solid evidence from other countries that lithium therapy had efficacy in bipolar disorder, and the FDA reversed its position and declared lithium as a treatment of choice for the condition. The USA was one of the last countries in the world to allow the medical use of lithium. Within a few years of lithium therapy, the number of hospitalized bipolar patients in the USA sharply dropped. Improved safety was achieved by exclusive use of lithium carbonate and through monitoring of lithium levels in blood. Lithium therapy has stood the test of time and continues as a leading bipolar therapy. I have met hundreds of patients who reported that lithium dramatically reduced their bipolar disorder symptoms. However, some lithium-treated patients experience severe kidney or liver problems and are forced to discontinue treatment. While many new psychiatric drugs have been developed for bipolar disorder, lithium remains as the initial treatment of choice in many parts of the world.

Lithium therapy can be very effective in combating mania but also results in far fewer hospitalizations during bipolar's depression phase. This has puzzled psychiatrists for years since lithium generally has very limited effectiveness during a depression episode. This is one of the mysteries examined in this study.

Clinical Insights and Adjunctive Therapies

In working with more than 1,500 bipolar patients over a 30-year period, my colleagues and I became familiar with the severe nature of the disorder and the limitations of today's mainstream and alternative treatments.[35] From our bipolar database of 200,000 blood/urine assays, we identified a high incidence of specific biochemical imbalances that appear to aggravate symptoms and make treatment more difficult. More than 95% in our bipolar population exhibited excessive reactive oxidative species (ROS) that can adversely affect brain function. Glutathione, catalase, metallothionein, and other natural antioxidants collaborate to reduce oxidative stress, but many individuals have an inborn genetic weakness in these protectors and may benefit from antioxidant supplements. As described in Chapter 8, genetic weakness in antioxidant protection appears to be a major predisposing factor in bipolar disorder. In addition, we found a high incidence of methylation disorders, zinc and B6 depletion, and copper overload that could significantly alter neurotransmission at serotonin, dopamine, norepinephrine (NE), N-methyl-D-aspartate (NMDA), and other receptor systems.[36] It seems unreasonable to ask psychiatric medications to cope with both bipolar disorder and unrelated chemical imbalances that may impair brain function. Adjunctive non-drug treatments for these comorbidities may improve efficacy of standard treatments for bipolar disorder.

Unique Features of Bipolar Disorder's Depression Phase

Throughout life, we all experience episodes of unhappiness, sadness, or grief that may occur when a loved one dies, or we suffer personal disappointment or tragedy. After a few weeks or months, most of us can recover and return to normal activities and mental outlook. This temporary depression is not a mental disorder, but rather an inevitable feature of human existence. However, other people experience clinical depression, a mental disorder associated with abnormal functioning of brain neurotransmitters.[18,37] Depression exists in all cultures and ethnic groups throughout the world. It strikes more than 50 million Americans, but only about 50% seek medical treatment. Typical symptoms include depressed mood, feelings of worthlessness or guilt, social withdrawal, agitation, problems with concentration, and difficulty sleeping. The severity of the condition may range from mild to severe. Millions are challenged by dysthymia, a relatively mild form of depression that involves sadness, lack of interest in daily activities, and feelings of inadequacy, which can persist for years. At the other end of the spectrum, major depressive disorder may involve severe psychic pain and thoughts of suicide.

Depression has existed since the beginning of recorded history. Hindu Vedas dating back to 1,500 B.C. emphasized the prevention of mental pain. The Old Testament describes King Saul's severe depression and ultimate suicide. Ancient civilizations thought depression was caused by evil spirits that could be released by drilling holes in the skull. In 440 B.C., Hippocrates dismissed this belief and insisted that depression must be explained by natural causes. In the next century, Plato erroneously revived the theory that depression was caused by mystical forces, but Aristotle later rejected this belief. The Roman philosopher Cicero theorized that depression resulted from life experiences and advocated a treatment similar to counseling. There was little progress in understanding this illness until the 19th century, when depression was recognized as a mental disorder and the medical and scientific communities actively sought effective therapies. Throughout the early 1900s, the predominant belief was that depression resulted from flawed or traumatic life experiences, especially in childhood. As described previously, talk therapies and counseling techniques dominated mainstream psychiatry until the mid-1960s when researchers learned the role of imbalanced NT systems; this gave birth to modern treatment approaches.[38] Within a few years, low serotonin neurotransmission became a focus of depression research. Early treatments were aimed at increasing brain levels of serotonin, also known as 5-hydroxytryptamine (5-HT), as well as combating monoamine oxidase (MAO) that metabolizes (removes) serotonin by chemical reaction. In the mid-1980s, scientists learned that serotonin activity was dominated by reuptake, a process in which 5-HT molecules are transported from a synapse back into the original presynaptic neuron. This led to the development of Prozac, Zoloft, and numerous other antidepressant medications that became the treatment of choice for depression throughout the world.

In recent years, scientists have learned that many cases of depression are unrelated to serotonin, and as a result, several novel medication therapies are under development. It is becoming clear that depression is an umbrella term used to describe a collection of disorders with quite different causes, symptoms, traits, and misbehaving NTs. In a study presented at the 2014 annual APA meeting,[39] my database of 300,000 blood/urine chemistry levels (2,800 unipolar non-bipolar depression patients) indicated the presence of five major phenotypes shown in Figure 1.

- Undermethylation was the largest chemical biotype (38%), with most patients reporting depression, anxiety, obsessive-compulsive disorder (OCD) tendencies, and perfectionism and a positive response to SSRI (selective serotonin reuptake inhibitor) antidepressants. Undermethylation of chromatin has been associated with elevated expression of serotonin transporter (SERT) reuptake proteins that reduce serotonin activity.
- Folate deficiency was the next largest biotype (20%), with most patients reporting high anxiety, sleep problems, food and chemical sensitivities, intolerance to SSRIs, and benefits from folate therapy or benzodiazepines.
- About 17% exhibited severe serum copper elevations associated with depressed dopamine and elevated norepinephrine. As seen in Figure 2, divalent copper (Cu^{++}) is a cofactor in synthesis of norepinephrine from dopamine. In two separate animal studies, abnormal serum copper levels had a massive effect on brain levels of these NTs. About 68% of ADHD patients and 95% of postpartum patients in my large chemical database exhibited very elevated serum copper levels.
- About 15% of our depressive population exhibited elevated urine pyrroles associated with severe oxidative stress and depressed zinc and B6 levels. Most pyrrole patients report extreme mood swings, fears, explosive anger, poor short-term memory, partial improvements from SSRIs, and major benefits from zinc and B6.
- A small depression phenotype (5%) involves overloads of lead, mercury, or other toxic metals. The remaining 5% shown in Figure 1 represents other forms of depression. Our data suggested that about 50% of our unipolar depression population exhibited low serotonin activity and were promising candidates for SSRI medication. The other depressives had distinctly different neurotransmission imbalances and symptomology.

Depression Biotypes

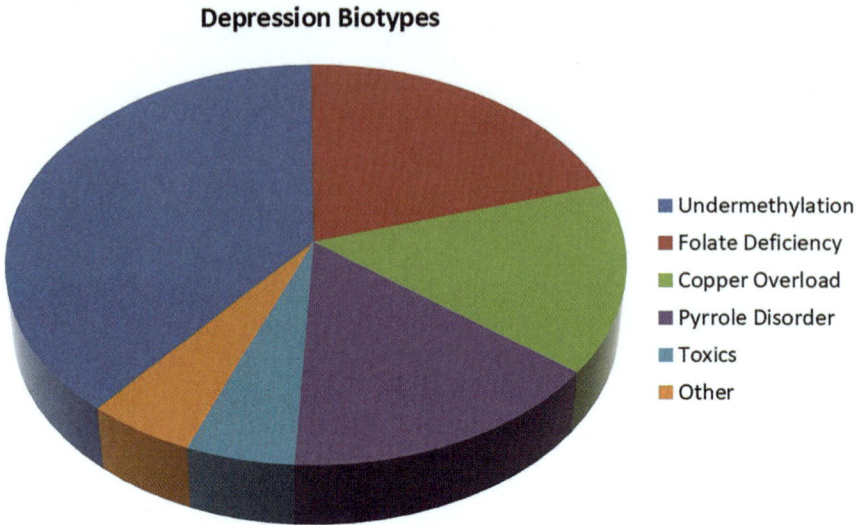

Figure 1. Biotypes of Clinical Depression

There are clear differences between typical clinical depressions and the depressive episodes experienced in bipolar disorder. For example, SSRI medications exhibit disappointing low efficacy during bipolar disorder's depression phase. This suggests that reuptake at serotonin receptors may not be a dominant feature of bipolar's depression phase. In addition, the transition from mania often involves sudden onset of severe depression that contrasts with the more gradual appearance of other mood disorders.

Most diagnosed bipolar 2 patients are especially challenged by transitions from hypomania to the despondency of severe depression and suicidal thoughts. Overall, it appears that the depression episodes encountered in bipolar disorders may involve different etiologies (causes) and unique misbehaving neurotransmitters compared to other mood disorders and psychotic conditions.

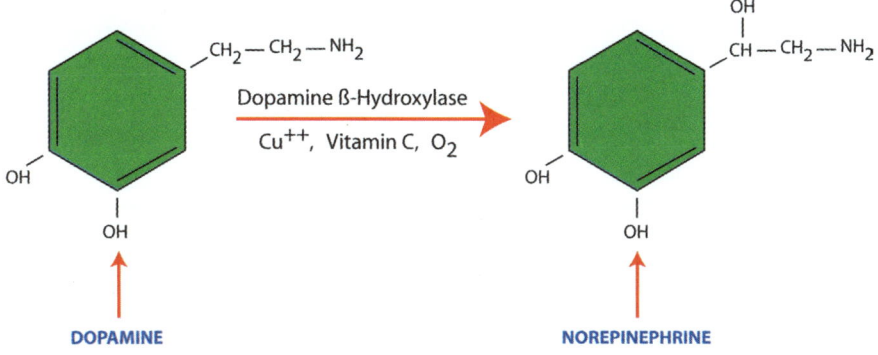

Figure 2. Synthesis of Norepinephrine from Dopamine

References

1.   Soares, J. C., & Young, A. H. (2016). *Bipolar disorders: Basic Mechanisms and Therapeutic Implications*. Cambridge University Press.

2.   Angst, J., & Marneros, A. (2001). Bipolarity from ancient to modern times: conception, birth and rebirth. *Journal of affective disorders*, *67*(1–3), 3–19.

3.   Falret, J. P. (1854). Mémoire sur la folie circulaire, forme de la maladie mentale caractérisée par la reproduction… Bulletin de l'Académie impériale de medicine. *Paris 1854; 19: 382, 400.*

4.   Kraepelin, E. (1919). Dementia praecox and paraphrenia. In G. M. Robertson (Ed), *Textbook of psychiatry 8th edition* (R. M. Barclay, Trans.). E. & S. Livingstone. (1896)

5.   Freud, S., & Strachey, J. (2007). *An outline of psycho-analysis* (Vol. 23). New York: Norton.

6.   Adler, A. (1992). *Understanding Human Nature* (C. Brett, Trans.). Oneworld Publications.

7.   Jung, C. G. (2024). *Collected Works of CG Jung, Volume 1: Psychiatric Studies* (Vol. 20). Princeton University Press.

8.   Wender, P. H., Kety, S. S., Rosenthal, D., Schulsinger, F., Ortmann, J., & Lunde, I. (1986). Psychiatric disorders in the biological and adoptive families of adopted individuals with affective disorders. *Archives of general psychiatry*, *43*(10), 923–929.

9.   Craddock, N., & Sklar, P. (2013). Genetics of bipolar disorder. *The Lancet*, *381*(9878), 1654–1662.

10. Bertelsen, A., Harvald, B., & Hauge, M. (1977). A Danish twin study of manic-depressive disorders. *The British Journal of Psychiatry, 130*(4), 330–351.

11. Katz, B. (1959). Mechanisms of synaptic transmission. *Reviews of Modern Physics, 31*(2), 524.

12. Axelrod, J. (1971). Noradrenaline: fate and control of its biosynthesis. *Science, 173*(3997), 598–606.

13. Rose, N. (2011). Historical changes in mental health practice. *Textbook of Community Mental Health.*

14. Goodman, L. S., Brunton, L. L., Chabner, B., & Knollmann, B. C. (2011). *Goodman & Gilman's Pharmacological Basis of Therapeutics* (12th ed.). McGraw-Hill.

15. Schatzberg, A. F., & Nemeroff, C. B. (2009). *The American psychiatric publishing textbook of psychopharmacology.* American Psychiatric Pub.

16. Hajda, M., Prasko, J., Latalova, K., Hruby, R., Ociskova, M., Holubova, M., ... & Mainerova, B. (2016). Unmet needs of bipolar disorder patients. *Neuropsychiatric disease and treatment*, 1561–1570.

17. Mondimore, F. M. (2014). *Bipolar disorder: A guide for patients and families* (3rd ed.). The Johns Hopkins University Press.

18. American Psychiatric Association: Diagnostic and Statistical Manual of Mental Disorders, Fifth Edition, Text Revision. Washington, DC, American Psychiatric Association, 2022.

19. Calabrese, J. R., Gao, K., & Sachs, G. (2017). Diagnosing Mania in the Age of DSM-5. *American Journal of Psychiatry, 174*(1), 8–10.

20. Freudenreich, O., Kontos, N., & Querques, J. (2012). Psychiatric polypharmacy: A clinical approach based on etiology and differential diagnosis. *Harvard Review of Psychiatry, 20*(2), 79–85.

21. Goldberg, J. F. (2019). Complex combination pharmacotherapy for bipolar disorder: knowing when less is more or more is better. *FOCUS, A Journal of the American Psychiatric Association, 17*(3), 218–231.

22. Zarate, C.A., Jr. and Quiroz, J.A. (2003), Combination treatment in bipolar disorder: a review of controlled trials. *Bipolar Disorders, 5*: 217–225.

23. Butler, M., Urosevic, S., Desai, P., Sponheim, S. R., Popp, J., Nelson, V. A., ... & Sunderlin, B. (2018). Treatment for bipolar disorder in adults: a systematic review.

24. Abrams, Z. (2020). Continuing education treating bipolar disorder in kids and teens. *Monitor on Psychology*, 41.

25. Stahl, S. M. (2008). *Depression and bipolar disorder: Stahl's essential psychopharmacology.* Cambridge University Press.

26. Slater, E., & Cowie, V. (1971). *The genetics of mental disorders.* Oxford U. Press.

27. Legrand, A., Iftimovici, A., Khayachi, A., & Chaumette, B. (2021). Epigenetics in bipolar disorder: a critical review of the literature. *Psychiatric genetics, 31*(1), 1–12.

28. D'addario, C., Dell'Osso, B., Palazzo, M. C., Benatti, B., Lietti, L., Cattaneo, E., ... & Altamura, A. (2012). Selective DNA methylation of BDNF promoter in bipolar disorder: differences among patients with BDI and BDII. *Neuropsychopharmacology, 37*(7), 1647–1655.

29. Jamison, K. R. (2019). Suicide and bipolar disorder. *Bipolar Disorder,* 115–119.

30. Jamison, K. R. (2000). Suicide and Bipolar Disorder. *Journal of Clinical Psychiatry, 61*(9), 47–51.

31. Pompili, M., Gonda, X., Serafini, G., Innamorati, M., Sher, L., Amore, M., ... & Girardi, P. (2013). Epidemiology of suicide in bipolar disorders: a systematic review of the literature. *Bipolar disorders, 15*(5), 457–490.

32. Cade, J. F. (1949). Lithium salts in the treatment of psychotic excitement. *Medical Journal of Australia.*

33. Shorter, E. (2009). The history of lithium therapy. *Bipolar disorders, 11,* 4–9.

34. Mitchell, P. B., & Hadzi-Pavlovic, D. (1999). John Cade and the discovery of lithium treatment for manic depressive illness. *Medical Journal of Australia, 171*(5), 262–264.

35. Cardoso, B. M., Dias, V. V., Frey, B. N., Gazalle, F. K., Kapczinski, F., & Kauer-Santa-Anna, M. (2010). Quality of life in bipolar disorder. *Handbook of Disease Burden and Quality of Life Measures,* 3591–3606.

36. Walsh, W. J. (2014). *Nutrient power.* Skyhorse Publishing.

37. Otte, C., Gold, S. M., Penninx, B. W., Pariante, C. M., Etkin, A., Fava, M., ... & Schatzberg, A. F. (2016). Major depressive disorder. *Nature reviews Disease primers, 2*(1), 1–20.

38. López-Muñoz, F., Bhatara, V. S., Alamo, C., & Cuenca, E. (2004). Historical approach to reserpine discovery and its introduction in psychiatry. *Actas espanolas de psiquiatria, 32*(6), 387–395.

39. Walsh, W.J. and deVito, R.A. (2014). "Chemical Biotypes of Depression and Individualized Nutrient Therapy." Annual APS Meeting: Research Abstracts. May 9, 2014. New York.

CHAPTER 2

A Search for the Essence
of Bipolar Disorder

Advances in Neuroscience

The past 30 years have seen great progress in identifying the intricate mechanisms of the human brain. Each tiny brain neuron is a highly complex hunk of protoplasm that accomplishes a great number of sophisticated functions. A major challenge in this study has been the extraordinary volume of new research findings published each month by neuroscientists throughout the world. Most of this research is basic in nature and not directed at individual brain disorders. I spent thousands of hours sifting through peer-reviewed abstracts and articles in a search for new research findings that might relate to bipolar disorder. Appendix D lists 287 scientific journals that were consulted during this investigation.

Recognizing that humans, animals, and insects share many identical genes and neuronal similarities, some of the greatest discoveries have involved lower forms of life. Knockout (deletion of single genes) mouse studies have identified the functional role of hundreds of human genes.[40] Early studies of scorpions and drosophila (fruit flies) led to pioneering understanding of potassium ion (K^+) channel behavior.[41] Squid giant axon research was a major event in neuroscience that brought the 1963 Nobel Prize to Hodgkin and Huxley for describing action potentials (the name given to neuron firing events) and the role of sodium ions.[42]

The development of microelectrode probes assisted early studies of membrane voltages and neuron behavior. A major breakthrough was the development of the patch-clamp method and single-channel recordings (1991 Nobel Prize to Neher and Sakmann).[43] This technique involves positioning tiny glass pipettes over single ion channels which allows measurement of ion flows across a neuron's membrane for different conditions. This system uses highly sensitive current to voltage convertors that accurately measure ion flow rates for microscopic single ion channels — a somewhat astonishing feat. Patch-clamp testing is very versatile and continues to be a mainstay of neuroscience experiments throughout the world.

Recent exponential progress in nanotechnology is providing neuroscientists with miniaturized probes, sensors, electrodes, and other instruments that enable previously unavailable testing of microscopic neurons. Advanced X-ray crystallographic techniques are defining the intricate substructure of axons, organelles, microtubules, vesicles, ion channels, myelin sheaths, and other neuronal components (described in detail in Chapter 3). Novel optogenetic techniques enable researchers to monitor and control neuronal activity with considerable precision using light signals. These are just a few examples of advances in nanotechnology that are enabling great progress in understanding of the brain.

Another breakthrough involves new synchrotron and other large particle accelerator machines that produce submicron-size X-ray beams for chemical or structural analysis of neurons, glial cells, and other microscopic brain components. In the early 2000s, I obtained access to Argonne National Laboratory's Advanced Photon Source (APS) for three experiments. My first APS adventure, lasting just six hours, assayed skull bone relics from composer Ludvig von Beethoven and revealed lead concentrations many times above toxic levels.[44] Two subsequent scouting experiments accurately assayed 14 elements in thin brain slices from deceased Alzheimer's disease, autism, and control subjects and provided a first glimpse at elemental concentrations at hundreds of locations in single neurons.[45] It's just a matter of time before chemical imbalances will be directly measured in neurons and glia for various disorders.

Epigenetic scientists are learning that misplaced or missing methyl imprints on deoxyribonucleic acid (DNA) can increase a risk for a mental disorder.[46,47] In 2022, Illinois researchers developed a technique for detecting methyl bookmarks on DNA locations in living persons using carbon-14 (radiocarbon) coupled with magnetic resonance imaging (MRI).[48] In addition, epigenetic research is identifying mechanisms by which emotional trauma, injury, or toxic exposures can damage DNA integrity and potentially trigger the onset of mental and physical disorders.[49,50]

For years, safety and ethics considerations severely restricted direct testing of a living person's brain, so most early research studies involved measurement of NT levels in blood, urine, and other periphery areas. Many years ago, I was excited to learn that more than 80% of our serotonin is not synthesized in the brain, but in the periphery of the body, and I started testing red blood cell membrane serotonin levels in criminals and mental patients. To my great disappointment, these levels completely failed to correlate with brain concentrations, and I forever abandoned this approach. In this investigation, all bipolar disorder studies based on peripheral serotonin, dopamine, or norepinephrine concentrations were considered highly suspect. Far more relevant have been cadaver studies and in vivo experiments that determine clinical response to medications that alter transmitter levels. For example, drugs that promote or inhibit reuptake can decrease or increase activity during mania, depression, or euthymia episodes. Many researchers study the impact of altering cytosol levels of a NT's precursor to evaluate the impact on mania or depression. Recent in vivo neuroimaging and functional magnetic resonance imaging studies are providing detailed information regarding the roles of serotonin, dopamine, and norepinephrine in bipolar disorder.[51]

Areas of Special Interest in Bipolar Disorder

Mania/Depression Cycling: The search for the cause and mechanisms of bipolar cycling has been a dominant activity throughout this study. Switching back and forth between depression and mania distinguishes bipolar disorder from all other psychiatric disorders.[52] Although this is a core aspect of the clinical presentation of the illness, I was unable to find convincing or plausible explanations in published literature. Medical research often provides answers to "what" before we learn "why." For example, scientists have identified brain areas and NT systems that exhibit altered functioning in bipolar disorder. In addition, differences in brain structure and connectivity associated with the illness have been discovered. Several studies[53] have explored responses to lithium and other psychiatric medications that might provide clues to the individual mania/depression transitions. Other studies have identified mutated genes, NT systems, medications, and other factors that have been implicated in cycling. Most of these factors deal with either a transition from mania to depression or depression to mania but fail to provide a plausible explanation for the chronic and often continuous mania/depression cycling that typically persists after bipolar disorder onset. This investigation searched neuroscience literature for possible insights regarding causes and mechanisms of this unique debilitating phenomenon.

Bipolar disorder represents a departure from relatively orderly and predictable brain function with the onset of alternating neuronal hyperactivity (mania) and hypoactivity (depression). I spent more than a year exploring conditions that could increase the rate of action potentials. Although actively debated in the literature, I came to believe that mania typically is dominated by hyperactivity at norepinephrine, dopamine, and glutamate, receptors,[54] while the misbehaving NTs responsible for bipolar depression phases are still unknown. I decided to study all aspects of neuronal functioning, with a focus on conditions that could disrupt regulation of neuron firing and neurotransmission. I was intrigued by the amazing ability of microscopic neurons to achieve very large resting voltages and fire up to 200 times each second. The amount of stored energy in the human brain is quite extraordinary and essential to proper function. Resting neuron voltages range between about 45 mV (millivolts) to 90 mV, with the majority operating around 70 mV. If only 20 of the brain's 80 billion neurons could be connected in series, they theoretically would attain the same voltage as a flashlight battery. The surprising high voltage of our microscopic neurons is essential to brain function, and lost ability to produce full resting potentials would likely result in mania. This and other possible causes of neuronal hyperactivity were a major aspect of this investigation.

Genetics Research: While the search for major bipolar genes was unsuccessful for decades, large genome-wide association studies (GWAS) have begun to identify low-effect genes associated with the disorder. It was announced in 2022 that all human DNA genes have been identified, and their most common (canonical) amino acid sequences have been determined. Genetic studies provide key information that improves our understanding of brain processes and the impacts of specific mutations. A mutation is defined as any departure from a gene's canonical sequence. This term is gradually being replaced by the expression gene variant since mutation has developed the connotation of a harmful change. In reality, DNA abnormalities may be beneficial, harmful, or have no effect. The greatest number of gene variants are single nucleotide polymorphisms (SNPs) in which a single nucleotide base is replaced by a different nucleotide base. For example, the risk of Alzheimer's disease is increased by a SNP in the instructions for an important biomolecule, which causes cysteine to be replaced by arginine.[55] Researchers have begun the process of identifying the functional role of all 20,000 genes and are learning the impact of individual SNP variants. However, the mechanistic role of many human genes is still unknown. For example, a multitude of transcription factors (TFs) and micro ribonucleic acid (microRNA or miRNA) genes that help regulate gene expression are poorly understood, and their variants might be important in bipolar disorder. Since bipolar disorder has a strong hereditary component but no prominent genes, it is apparent that impairment of many low-effect genes collaborates to produce this unique disorder. More than five dozen bipolar-related genes have already been identified, and the number seems to increase every year. This is a fertile area of research that may lead to the causes and detailed mechanisms of this complex and unique disorder.

Epigenetics and Loss of DNA Integrity: From the moment of birth, every DNA molecule experiences severe damage that is not completely repaired. This is why we gradually age with each advancing year. DNA orchestrates production of thousands of special proteins necessary for survival of every cell. The declining quality of expressed proteins is responsible for wrinkled skin and other physical changes but also is a major factor in late-onset mental disorders such as bipolar disorder. Cumulative emotional, chemical, or physical trauma can trigger epigenetic changes that may be permanent.

I decided to explore hypothetical epigenetic events that might lead to the onset of bipolar disorder. Of special interest are unrepaired DNA damage, environmental insults, and epigenetic changes that could cause the persistent neuronal hyperactivity associated with mania typically observed during bipolar onset. Recognizing that the switch to depression usually occurs after increasing mania severity, I examined the possibility that *persistent extreme mania is the actual cause of the depression phase.* For example, sustained rapid neuronal firing might overwhelm vulnerable brain areas and lead to local loss of function. This investigation also assessed possible temporary impairment of the raphe nuclei that distribute serotonin throughout the brain, since this might explain the chronic appearance and disappearance of the depression phase in bipolar disorder.

Epigenetics and Unification of Psychiatry Paradigms: Epigenetics is gradually leading to unification of two competing schools of thought in psychiatry. For many decades, mainstream psychiatry believed that most mental illnesses are primarily caused by severe trauma, especially in childhood. This led to elaborate counseling and talk therapy approaches aimed at helping patients challenged by anxiety, depression, and other mental disorders. Since 1950, other psychiatrists have concentrated on receptors, NTs, and molecular biology of the brain. For many years, the two camps have had little regard for each other's beliefs. However, recent epigenetic studies indicate that emotional trauma can alter gene expression and permanently impair neurotransmission, suggesting that both approaches have validity and are complementary. I'm reminded of lyrics in a song from *Oklahoma!*, "The farmer and the cowboy should be friends."

Lithium Efficacy Theories: Although lithium therapy has benefited millions of bipolar patients since Cade's accidental discovery in the 1940s, psychiatry remains uncertain about the mechanisms of improvement. Approximately one-third of bipolar patients treated with lithium report major improvement, another one-third exhibit partial reduction of symptoms, and the remainder essentially fail to improve.[56] Lithium is a micronutrient present in all humans at extremely low concentrations, and there is considerable evidence that relatively low natural levels in the body are associated with depression, suicide, and criminal behavior. I first encountered this in forensic studies of prison residents in the 1970s. In collaboration with world-class chemists at Argonne National Laboratory, I found a strong inverse relationship between scalp-hair Li levels and degree of violence. Death row inmates and other convicted murderers at Illinois' Stateville Correctional Center exhibited Li levels below 0.01 ppb (parts per billion), compared to 0.02–0.04 ppb for other inmates, and greater than 0.06 ppb for age-matched controls. This correlated with the Amarillo findings described in Chapter 1. Today, there is general agreement that abnormally low Li levels are associated with a higher risk for mental problems.

Standard lithium therapy for bipolar disorder increases blood levels far beyond natural levels. The therapeutic range for lithium has been established at 0.6–1.2 mmol/L (millimoles per liter) in serum. Within this narrow range, most patients will respond to the drug without symptoms of toxicity. Periodic blood testing is required to maintain Li levels at safe levels. The most serious side effects involve kidney or liver damage in highly sensitive individuals. For years, researchers have studied lithium's impact on brain function looking for clues that might reveal the cause and mechanisms of bipolar disorder. This has resulted in several plausible explanations for lithium's effectiveness that are still being debated.[57] Very high therapeutic lithium levels impact many aspects of human biochemistry including the following:

- Improved immune function involving granulocytosis, lymphopenia, and natural killer cells (NK cells).
- Inhibition of glycogen synthase kinase-3 beta (GSK-3β)
- Up-regulation of brain-derived neurotrophic factor (BDNF) and other factors that regulate growth and synapse formation.
- Stimulation of neuronal stem cells.
- Increased brain levels of myo-inositol and N-acetylaspartate (NAA).
- Protection of neurons against glutamate excesses, seizures, and neurotoxins.
- Competition with sodium ions (Na^+) as both rush through voltage-gated channels during initiation of action potentials.
- Increased expression of the ADCY2 gene (an early GWAS variant for bipolar disorder) that catalyzes production of cyclic AMP that is crucial for many neuronal functions.

My arbitrary belief is that lithium's efficacy for bipolar disorder is most likely due to one of the following: (a) GSK-3 inhibition, (b) competition between influx of Li^+ and Na^+ ions during neuron firing, or (c) an abnormal expression of ADCY2. In any case, lithium studies remain a fertile area for bipolar research since detailed knowledge of its impact on brain function may eventually reveal important aspects of this still mysterious disorder.

Oxidative Stress and Bipolar Disorder: There is strong consensus among neuroscientists that elevated oxidative stress is a major feature of most bipolar disorders. As mentioned in the previous chapter, more than 95% of our 1,500 bipolar patients exhibited major oxidative overload. This suggests that free-radical assaults on DNA may be accelerating the loss of DNA integrity, especially in persons with genetically weakened gene teams that regulate neuronal firing rates. Another possibility is that individuals prone to bipolar disorder may have genetic impairments in expression of glutathione peroxidase, catalase, superoxide dismutase (SOD), or other antioxidant genes needed to protect DNA against environmental or internal sources of free radicals. Every DNA strand in our body develops between 10,000 and a million lesions every day that require repair. It would be very surprising if genetically weakened DNA protection didn't contribute to bipolar predisposition. In addition, most of our patients reported significant partial clinical improvement after antioxidant therapy, suggesting that oxidative overload is a continuing barrier to clinical improvement after onset of the disorder. An important question is whether antioxidant supplements could reduce the risk of developing bipolar disorder.

Ion Channels: Any study of neuronal behavior and neurotransmission must involve the complex behavior of sodium, potassium, calcium, and chlorine ion channels embedded in our neuronal membranes. Sodium-potassium pumps (also called Na^+/K^+-ATPase or Na^+/K^+ pumps) create large ion gradients across neuronal membranes that produce the instability needed for action potentials. Leak channels produce resting potentials, and voltage-gated channels enable neuron firing events. Abnormal ion channel behavior is a leading suspect in neuronal hyperactivity or hypoactivity and was intensively studied throughout this investigation (see Chapter 4).

Glial Cells: Human brains have billions of glial cells that provide structural support for fragile brain neurons. After a century of neglect, scientists were surprised to learn that glial cells actually have many critical roles in neurotransmission and are now the subject of intensive research throughout the world. Astrocyte and oligodendrocyte glia assist regulation of neuronal activity, and glia impairments are likely contributors to the etiology of bipolar disorder.

Summary: The first two years of study identified the above aspects of brain function as especially promising in the search for the cause and mechanisms of bipolar disorder. Recent neuroscience progress has been explosive, and many cherished beliefs seem headed for the wastebasket. Scientists are learning the important roles of ion channel impairments, epigenetic changes, altered methyl bookmarking, DNA repair mechanisms, transcription factors, microRNA regulation of gene expression, alternative splicing, and a host of other key factors in mental illnesses. Much of this information has not yet impacted clinical treatment. We are in the early stages of a revolution in brain science that will lead to improved therapies and, perhaps, the effective prevention of bipolar disorder.

References

40. Hall, B., Limaye, A., & Kulkarni, A. B. (2009). Overview: generation of gene knockout mice. *Current protocols in cell biology, 44*(1), 19–12.

41. Swartz, K. J. (2013). The scorpion toxin and the potassium channel. *Elife, 2,* e00873.

42. Schwiening, C. J. (2012). A brief historical perspective: Hodgkin and Huxley. *The Journal of physiology, 590*(Pt 11), 2571.

43. Neher, E., & Sakmann, B. (1992). The patch clamp technique. *Scientific American, 266*(3), 44–51.

44. Weinstein, L. (Director). (2005). *Beethoven's Hair* [Film]. British Broadcasting Corporation.

45. Walsh, W.J., Lai, B., Bazan, N., & Lukiw, W.L. (2005). Trace metal analysis in Alzheimer's disease tissues using high brilliance X-Ray beams. In *Fifth Keele Meeting on Trace Metals and Neurotoxicity in the Brain,* Department of Biology University of Aveiro, Portugal.

46. Keverne, E. B., Pfaff, D. W., & Tabansky, I. (2015). Epigenetic changes in the developing brain: Effects on behavior. *Proceedings of the National Academy of Sciences, 112*(22), 6789–6795.

47. Nestler, E. J., Peña, C. J., Kundakovic, M., Mitchell, A., & Akbarian, S. (2016). Epigenetic basis of mental illness. *The Neuroscientist, 22*(5), 447–463.

48. Lam, F., Chu, J., Choi, J. S., Cao, C., Hitchens, T. K., Silverman, S. K., ... & Li, K. C. (2022). Epigenetic MRI: noninvasive imaging of

DNA methylation in the brain. *Proceedings of the National Academy of Sciences, 119*(10), e2119891119.

49. Young, A. H., & Juruena, M. F. (2021). The neurobiology of bipolar disorder. In *Bipolar Disorder: From Neuroscience to Treatment* (pp. 1–20). Cham: Springer International Publishing.

50. Selye, H. (1973). The Evolution of the Stress Concept: The originator of the concept traces its development from the discovery in 1936 of the alarm reaction to modern therapeutic applications of syntoxic and catatoxic hormones. *American scientist, 61*(6), 692–699.

51. Ching, C. R., Hibar, D. P., Gurholt, T. P., Nunes, A., Thomopoulos, S. I., Abé, C., ... & ENIGMA Bipolar Disorder Working Group. (2022). What we learn about bipolar disorder from large-scale neuroimaging: Findings and future directions from the ENIGMA Bipolar Disorder Working Group. *Human brain mapping, 43*(1), 56–82.

52. Salvadore, G., Quiroz, J. A., Machado-Vieira, R., Henter, I. D., Manji, H. K., & Zarate Jr, C. A. (2010). The neurobiology of the switch process in bipolar disorder: a review. *The Journal of clinical psychiatry, 71*(11), 12633.

53. Ochoa, E. L. (2022). Lithium as a neuroprotective agent for bipolar disorder: an overview. *Cellular and molecular neurobiology, 42*(1), 85–97.

54. Manji, H. K., Quiroz, J. A., Payne, J. L., Singh, J., Lopes, B. P., Viegas, J. S., & Zarate, C. A. (2003). The underlying neurobiology of bipolar disorder. *World Psychiatry, 2*(3), 136.

55. Saunders, A. M., Schmader, K., Breitner, J. C., Benson, M. D., Brown, W. T., Goldfarb, L., ... & McCown, N. (1993). Apolipoprotein E epsilon 4 allele distributions in late-onset Alzheimer's disease and in other amyloid-forming diseases. *Lancet (London, England), 342*(8873), 710–711.

56. Rakofsky, J. J., Lucido, M. J., & Dunlop, B. W. (2022). Lithium in the treatment of acute bipolar depression: A systematic review and meta-analysis. *Journal of affective disorders, 308*, 268–280.

57. Malhi, G. S., Tanious, M., Das, P., Coulston, C. M., & Berk, M. (2013). Potential mechanisms of action of lithium in bipolar disorder: Current understanding. *CNS drugs, 27*(2), 135–153.

CHAPTER 3

The Amazing Neuron

Neurons are cells that receive, process, and transmit electrochemical signals at speeds up to 200 mph. Our brains contain between 60 to 90 billion neurons as well as a similar number of glial cells. Neurons were discovered in the early 1800s by Jan Evangelista Purkinje,[58] Carmillo Golgi,[59] and others using tissue-staining chemicals and high-magnification microscopes. Originally, they assumed that brain neurons were directly connected, forming a complicated electrical circuit. Over the next 30 years, extraordinary progress in brain science was achieved despite the primitive equipment available at the time. In the 1880s, Spanish scientist Ramon y Cajal[60] discovered that neurons didn't actually touch, but instead they communicated by sending signals to nearby neurons. Ramon y Cajal believed that the signals were electrical sparks that jumped from neuron to neuron. In the 1890s, Charles Sherrington in England[61] discovered that communication between neurons was chemical in nature and occurred across a tiny gap between brain cells that he called a "synapse," from the Greek word meaning "to clasp."

Two hundred years of intensive study has revealed the elaborate configuration and great complexity of these microscopic cells.[62] Like snowflakes, no two brain neurons are exactly alike. They vary in size from 4 microns to 100 microns in diameter and from about 250 microns to 10,000 microns in length. Figures 3 and 4 are schematic drawings that show the major component parts of a neuron.

Each brain neuron is enclosed in a bilayer lipid membrane that prevents external fluids from entering the cell.[63] The plasma membrane is an excellent insulator that provides electrical isolation from other neurons. It is embedded with Ca, Na, K, and Cl ion channels and Na/K pumps that confer an electrochemical potential and excitability to the membrane. Most neurons develop a resting voltage of about -70 mV. However, membrane potential constantly changes as NTs from nearby neurons interact with dendrite receptors to open pores and allow inward flow of excitatory or inhibitory ions. If threshold voltage (about -55 mV) is reached, the neuron will fire NTs into a synapse. A bilayer membrane's capacitor-like storage of electrical charge provides some of the impetus for action potentials. Neuronal membranes are not lifeless and passive but actively control the passage of gases, nutrients, and waste products into and out of the cell.

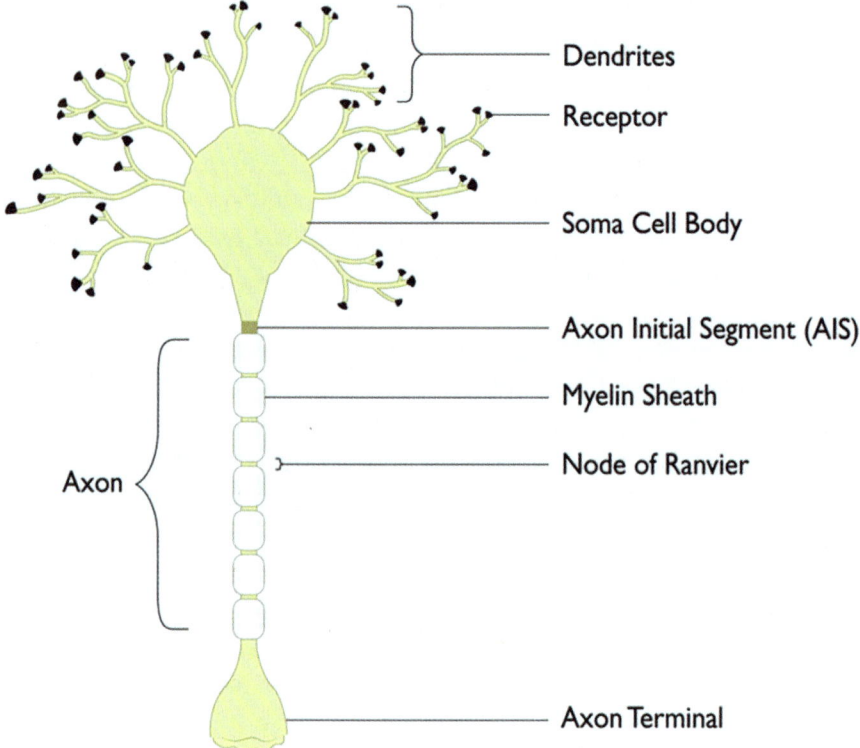

Figure 3. Schematic Drawing of a Neuron

The Soma Cell Body

This large roughly spherical part of the neuron contains the same component parts (organelles) found in other human cells and performs similar functions including energy production and protein synthesis. However, a neuronal soma also has branching dendrites (signal receivers) and a long wire-like projection called an axon that conducts nerve signals to its terminal where NTs are released into synapses. Most somas contain a centrally located spherical nucleus of about 5–10 micrometers diameter that contains DNA double-helix molecules that are encased in a membrane called the nuclear envelope. Key soma organelles are described below:

- *Cytoplasm*: Cytoplasm refers to the interior contents of a neuron, not including the nucleus. The cytoskeleton, which has a framework of protein scaffolds, enables the fragile neuron to retain its shape. The cytoskeleton and cytosol liquid form a thick jelly-like material that completely fills the neuron's vacant spaces. The nucleus, ribosomes, mitochondria, and other organelles are suspended and remain in place to perform their specialized functions. In addition, cytoplasm stores molecules required for cellular processes and assists in removal of trash.
- *Nucleus*: Each neuron's DNA contains about 20,000 coding genes that coordinate the production of enzymes, ion channels, vesicles, microtubules, and other neuronal components. The double-helix DNA is trapped within the nuclear envelope, but single-stranded mRNA (messenger ribonucleic acid) molecules can pass through tiny pores to access the reticulum-ribosome organelles for production of expressed proteins. The nuclear envelope shields the genome from cytoplasm components and provides anchoring sites for chromatin and cytoskeleton.
- *Mitochondria*: Several thousand of these sausage-shaped structures are present in each cell in the body, including neuronal cells. Their job is to process oxygen and convert the foods we consume into energy. This involves cellular respiration in which the complex Krebs cycle produces adenosine triphosphate (ATP) that provides 90% of the body's energy. Mitochondrial ATP provides the energy for sodium-potassium pumps to establish ion gradients across neuronal membranes and form resting voltages that are essential to neurotransmission. Importantly, there is scientific evidence that mitochondrial function is impaired in bipolar disorder, and many researchers have theorized this as the primary cause of the condition. I spent months

studying this possibility but was unable to find a mitochondrial connection with mania/depression cycling. However, mitochondrial energy production is a major source of ROS including superoxide and other free radicals associated with inflammation and DNA damage in bipolar disorder.[63,64]

- *Ribosomes*: These complex molecules contain ribosomal RNA (rRNA) and specialized proteins and are the site for protein synthesis. Each ribosome has a subunit that reads a protein's genetic code from the mRNA template and another subunit that assembles the corresponding amino acids to form the appropriate protein. Ribosomes are mitten-shaped and attach to walls of reticulum structures where expressed proteins are produced in a process called translation. In essence, ribosomes use the blueprint provided by mRNA to assemble needed proteins.

- *Rough endoplasmic reticulum* (RER): This membranous organelle adjacent to the nucleus is studded with ribosomes that provide a rough appearance. In essence, the RER and its associated ribosomes represent the cell's protein production machinery. In addition, RER assists in synthesis, folding, modification, and transport of new proteins.

- *Smooth endoplasmic reticulum* (SER): This membrane-bound network of tubules does not contain ribosomes, which is why it has a smooth appearance. The SER is the site for synthesis of lipids, steroids, and carbohydrates and is located away from the cell's nucleus.

- *Microtubules*: Microtubules, together with microfilaments and intermediate filaments, form the neuron's cytoskeleton. They are involved in mitosis (cell division), cell motility, transport of vesicles and enzymes down the axon (axonal transport), and maintenance of cell shape.

- *Golgi apparatus*: This soma organelle stores and modifies new proteins produced in ribosomes for special functions and prepares them for transport to specific neuron locations. For example, the Golgi apparatus modifies new enzymes and vesicles that attach to tiny axon microtubules for transport to the terminal bulb area where NTs are synthesized.

- *Lysosomes*: The main function of these cell organelles is the digestion and removal of unwanted cell components and debris. The lysosomes contain 40 separate hydrolases capable of degrading proteins, lipids, and carbohydrates. Using water, hydrolases are in a class of enzymes that break down molecules into smaller molecules.

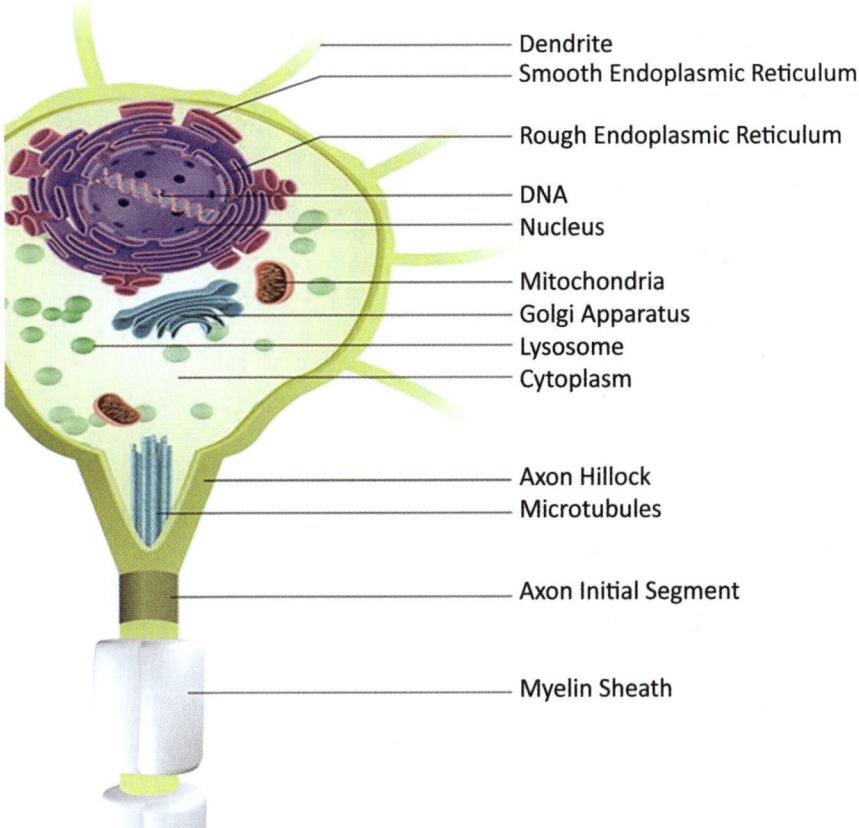

Figure 4. The Neuron's Soma Cell Body

Dendrites

These membrane projections receive NT signals from nearby neurons across a synapse. They contain special ion channels that open after contact with a specific NT, causing inhibitory or excitatory ions to enter the neuron and alter the membrane's potential (voltage). Some large neurons have more than 10,000 dendrites that form a tree-like conformation, while others have just a few dozen dendrites (see

Figure 5). In addition to signal reception, they also can form spikes that assist long-term potentiation (LTP), a process that strengthens brain neuron connections that enable memory.

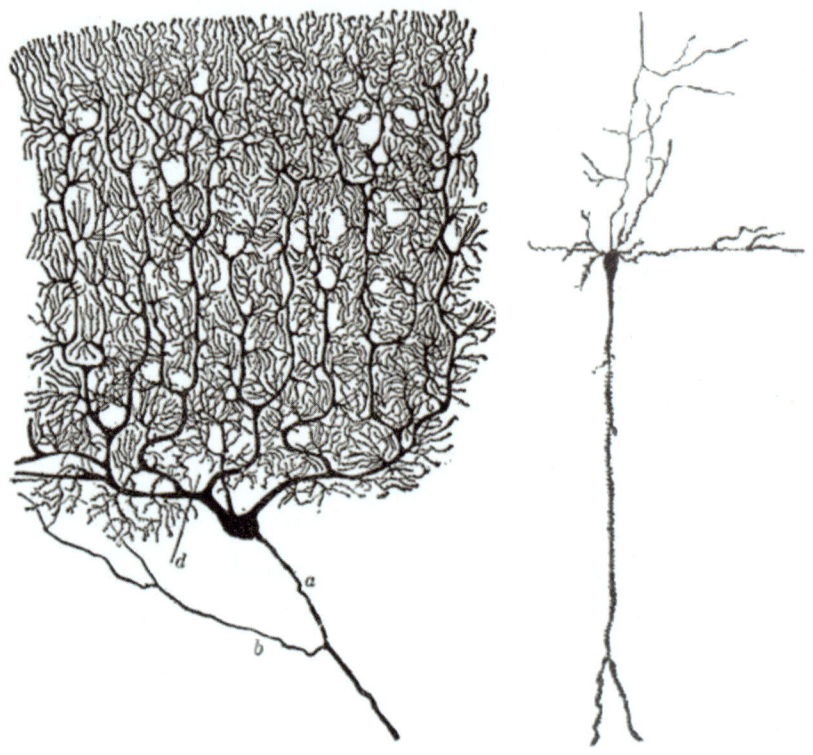

Figure 5. Dendritic Tree Variations in Neurons

The Axon

Most brain neurons have a thin cable-like projection called an axon that extends from the soma to the synaptic terminal. Axons vary in length from a few micrometers to several centimeters. Their diameter is usually constant until approaching its terminus where the axon may (or may not) branch into several projections that can terminate at separate synaptic clefts.

The Axon Initial Segment (AIS) Control Center: The control center for a brain neuron is the AIS.[65] The AIS is located on the edge of the axon hillock, a conical bridge from soma to axon. The AIS has no myelin coating and contains a multitude of voltage-gated Na^+ channels that are normally closed. The AIS determines the voltage impacts from the neuron's many receptors and senses the overall voltage at each point in time. If AIS threshold voltage is reached, its Na^+ channels spring open to trigger a voltage pulse that travels down to the axon terminus and initiates release of NTs into a synapse. The AIS has a high degree of plasticity and can alter its physical shape and distribution of ion channels in response to a changing environment.

Myelin and the Nodes of Ranvier: Most of the axon is coated with a myelin sheath (an insulating layer) that prevents leakage of ions as the voltage pulse travels down the axon. However, axons have gaps in the myelin called nodes of Ranvier that are exposed to the extra-cellular fluid (see Figure 3). The nodes contain extraordinary concentrations of voltage-gated Na^+ channels that assist in transmitting a voltage pulse. The nodes act as voltage boosters when the action potential reaches them by opening their voltage-gated Na^+ channels. In this way, the voltage pulse jumps from node to node until it reaches the axon terminus and initiates neurotransmission. The myelin coating is composed of specialized glial cells that are described in Chapter 5.

The Axon Terminus: The cytoplasm fluid within the axon terminus contains numerous vesicles filled with NTs. Some of the vesicles float freely in cytoplasm while others are docked at the presynaptic membrane in preparation for ejection of NTs into a synapse. When an action potential pulse reaches the terminus, voltage-gated Ca^{++} channels open, and the inrush of Ca^{++} ions triggers the release of NTs into the synapse by a process called exocytosis.

Neuron Longevity: Brain neurons are the most durable cells in the human body. The average adult has about 37 trillion cells including an estimated 80 billion neurons. Most of our body's cells have a limited lifetime and are regularly replaced by cell division (called mitosis). In contrast, neurons do not divide and exhibit remarkable longevity. If we live beyond 100 years, most of our neurons will be the same ones that have served us since birth. This is especially surprising since every neuron's DNA is assaulted daily by cosmic radiation, oxidative stress, and other insults that produce single-strand DNA breaks, double-strand breaks, and harmful chemical reactions. DNA repair processes (described in Chapter 6 and Appendix B) are among the most complex and amazing attributes of the human body. In addition, the neuron's longevity is enhanced by the blood-brain barrier (BBB) that limits the access of toxins and other sources of oxidative stress. Also, the skull attenuates some of the cosmic radiation that can damage DNA. Unfortunately, DNA repair is not able to overcome every insult. It is estimated that healthy young adults lose about 31 million brain neurons each year, corresponding to a loss of 1% every 26 years. This suggests the potential for high cognitive function well beyond 100 years if we learn how to minimize neuron loss as we age.

The Neurotransmitter Life Cycle

Neurotransmitters are chemical messengers that enable brain neurons to communicate with each other. In 1921, Austrian scientist Otto Loewi discovered the first NT, now known as acetylcholine.[66] He became famous after recounting that his prize-winning experiment occurred to him in a dream. Since then, over 40 neurotransmitters have been identified in the human brain. My investigation concentrated on serotonin, dopamine, norepinephrine, glutamate, and GABA since impairments in these NT systems are associated with the most common mental disorders.

We are not born with a lifetime supply of these NTs. Instead, they are continuously produced by chemical reactions in brain cells and after a period of service are chemically degraded. The life cycle steps are synthesis, packaging into vesicles, ejection into a synapse, interactions with nearby neurons, followed by either deactivation by enzymes or reuptake into its original neuron home.[67] Most NTs are synthesized in the cytoplasm of presynaptic terminals and transported into vesicles. In an exception, norepinephrine is directly synthesized within vesicles. The reactants are amino acids and other molecules that enter the neuron through the glial cell network. Enzymes for the reaction are genetically expressed in the ribosomes and Golgi apparatus and travel the long journey to the axon terminus. After synthesis, the NTs are stored in tiny vesicles[68] which resemble tiny bubbles swimming in the cell liquid (cytosol). Like enzymes, vesicles are formed in ribosomes and Golgi apparatus and travel to the terminus. Approximately 200 NTs may be loaded into each vesicle through transport proteins called vesicular monoamine transporters (VMATs)[24] embedded in vesicle membranes. Some of the "loaded" vesicles attach to the neuron's membrane at docking sites where NTs can be launched into the synapse.

When a brain cell fires (action potential), Ca^{++} ions rush into the cell, causing vesicles to fuse with the plasma membrane, allowing NT molecules to be sprayed into the synapse. The vesicle residues are either absorbed into the cell membrane or returned to the cytosol for formation of new vesicles. A fraction of the NT molecules travel across the synapse to receptors of postsynaptic cells and transmit a chemical message that either promotes or inhibits cell firing. For example, activating a glutamate receptor is excitatory and tends to promote firing. In contrast, docking at a GABA receptor is calming and tends to inhibit an action potential. After a brief interaction, the NT molecule is released from the receptor back into the synapse.

Neurotransmitters released into a synapse tend to be quickly returned to the original cell through transmembrane proteins in a process called reuptake. The returning NTs are packaged into new vesicles for reuse. In the 1980s, we learned that reuptake dominates NT activity, and it is now the target of most depression medications. For example, SSRI antidepressants interfere with expression of SERT proteins, slowing the reuptake process, enabling serotonin neurotransmissions for a prolonged period. Some NTs undergo chemical degradation in the synapse before they can return to the parent neuron. For example, monoamine oxidase reacts with a fraction of synaptic serotonin and removes them from the scene. In addition, some NT molecules diffuse away from the synapse and are lost by that mechanism.

Neurotransmission

Figure 6 illustrates the communication between brain neurons. A neuron that sends a signal across a synapse is called presynaptic, and a neuron that receives the signal is termed postsynaptic. When a neuron fires, an electrochemical pulse is sent down the axon to the terminus, releasing NT molecules into the synaptic space. Some of these NTs link with receptors of nearby cells, sending an activating or inhibiting signal to those cells. This is the basic way in which brain cells communicate with each other. If a sufficient number of brain cells are activated, a thought or action can result.

Receptors[69] are genetically expressed ion channels embedded in neuron membranes that open when activated by a specific NT. Most receptors have a unique configuration that can receive a signal from only one type of NT. For example, a serotonin receptor may be activated only by a serotonin molecule. In ionotropic receptors, activation causes the receptor to twist like a contortionist to form a pore that allows ions to enter or leave the neuron. In contrast, metabotropic G-protein-coupled receptors (GPCRs) respond to NT activation by sending a second messenger molecule that opens a pore in the neuron's membrane. A single neuron may have thousands of dendrite receptors that interact with glutamate, serotonin, GABA, or other NTs, causing an intermittent inrush of excitatory or inhibitory ions that continuously alter neuron voltage.

The Action Potential: An action potential[70] is an explosive surge in a neuron's membrane voltage that culminates in spraying of NTs into a synapse. Figure 7 is a schematic drawing that shows the voltage changes during different stages of an action potential.

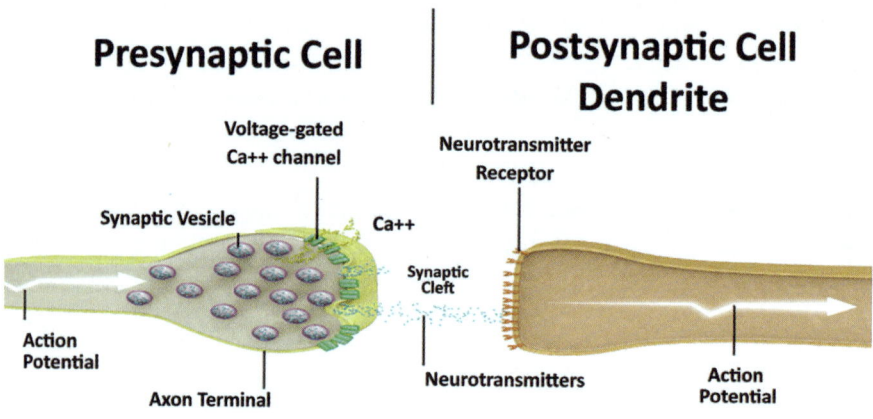

Figure 6. Communication between Brain Neurons

When a neuron's threshold voltage is reached, voltage-gated Na$^+$ ions spring open and trigger an unstoppable chain of events that result in neuron firing followed by return to the original condition.

Step 1: The neuron's initial resting voltage is established.
Step 2: Neurotransmitter voltage inputs are summed at the AIS.
Step 3: If threshold voltage is reached, voltage-gated Na$^+$ ion channels open, and the inward ion flow causes membrane voltage to suddenly change from negative to positive.

Step 4: The voltage pulse travels to the axon terminus where it opens Ca⁺⁺ channels.

Step 5: The inrush of Ca⁺⁺ ions causes neurotransmitters to enter a synapse.

Step 6: At peak voltage, the gated Na⁺ channels shut, and K⁺ channels open to enable a rapid return to the resting voltage (repolarization).

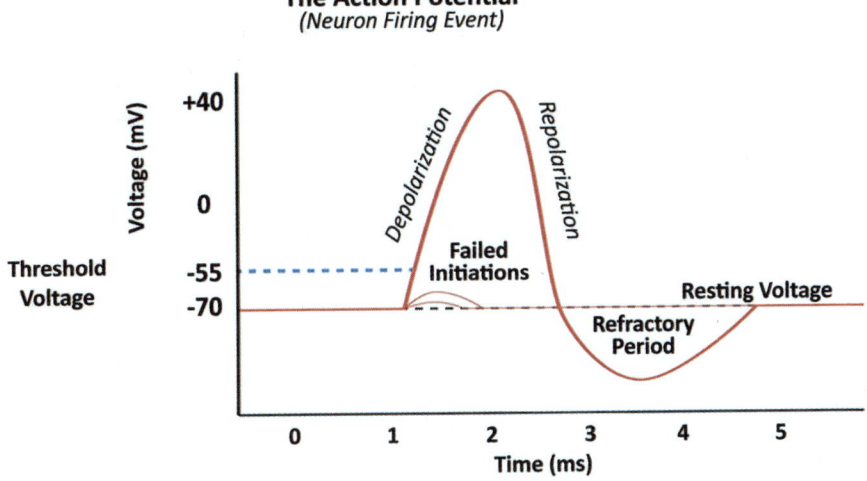

Figure 7. The Action Potential

Resting Voltages and Polarity: Each neuron develops a surprisingly large voltage despite its microscopic size. The resting voltage depends on ion gradients across the membrane and ion flows across leak channels (described in Chapter 4 and Appendix A). Despite the high K⁺ concentration within the neuron, the cytosol has a negative charge due to its large phosphate ion content. By convention, the resting voltage is termed negative. When a neuron fires, voltage becomes positive temporarily due to the rapid inflow of Na⁺ ions. The rapid return to negative rest voltage is aided by rapid outflow of K⁺ ions during repolarization. Neuroscientists have identified the complex mechanisms for each phase of an action potential, including the return to the resting state. This remarkable sequence is accomplished in just a few milliseconds. The choreography of neuron firing is as elegant and coordinated as a Fred Astaire dance routine.

Receptor Activity Impacts Neuron Voltage: As shown in Figure 5, individual neurons have great variations in the number of dendrites and receptors. A receptor is essentially an ion channel embedded in a neuron's membrane that receives NT signals from nearby neurons. A large neuron may have more than a thousand dendrites and a wide variety of receptor types. When an NT from a nearby neuron docks at a receptor, specific ions flow into the postsynaptic neuron producing a change in overall membrane voltage. For example, neurotransmission at glutamate receptors opens ion channels that produce inward flow of Na^+ and Ca^{++} ions, causing voltage to approach the firing threshold. GABA, the brain's primary calming NT, inhibits cell firing through the inward flow of chloride ions (Cl^-) that move voltage farther from threshold. If excitatory neurotransmission dominates, membrane voltage may reach threshold and initiate an action potential. The NTs released may or may not activate receptors of other neurons and influence their behavior.

A key aspect of bipolar disorder is impaired regulation of neuronal activity and onset of chronic oscillation between mania and depression. This investigation was keenly interested in possible causes and mechanisms of this unique late-onset loss of stability. As previously mentioned, many patients are capable of high achievement despite the severe challenges of bipolar disorder, and it is likely that parts of the brain may function normally, while other sites may be impaired.

Neurotransmitter Clearance from Receptors: While the action potential races down the axon at speeds up to 200 mph, a comparatively slower voltage pulse travels across the soma and dendritic tree. This releases NTs still attached at receptors and closes the receptors' ion channel pores. Within 5–10 milliseconds, the neuron is ready for the next action potential. Neuron firing events are limited to about 200 per second by the brief refractory periods during repolarization when action potentials are impossible before the earlier ones fade away.

Neurotransmission, Graded Potentials, and Summation: A neurotransmitter docking at a receptor generally changes membrane potential by less than one mV. Numerous receptors must be activated to cause neuron firing, since threshold voltage may be 10–25 mV from the resting voltage. Summation is a term used to describe the net voltage at the AIS, resulting from the combination of excitatory and inhibitory NTs. The impact of a single receptor-activation depends on its timing and distance from the AIS. If the net membrane voltage is insufficient to cause the neuron to fire, the momentary voltage is referred to as a graded potential, which quickly fades away. Temporal summation refers to the additive effect of several graded potentials that occur at a synapse so rapidly that they build on each other before the early ones fade. Spatial summation refers to the combined voltage effect from simultaneously activated nearby synapses.

Voltage Changes during Neuron Firing: When a neuron fires, the inrush of Na^+ ions suddenly changes membrane voltage from negative to positive, as seen in Figure 7. When the voltage pulse reaches the axon terminus, voltage-gated Ca^{++} channels open causing NTs to spray into the synapse. After only about one millisecond, all the Ca^{++} and Na^+ voltage-gated channels close, returning K^+ permeability to dominance and sending voltage back to the rest potential. Some calcium-activated potassium channels remain open temporarily during repolarization to accelerate the neuron's return to the original condition. As seen in Figure 7, the voltage briefly drops below the resting potential during repolarization until these channels close. It's quite remarkable that nearly all of our 80 billion individual tiny neurons are capable of this complex choreography.

Neuronal Hyperactivity and Bipolar Mania

The sine qua non characteristic of bipolar disorder is a history of one or more episodes of mania that is associated with generalized neuronal hyperactivity. I decided to (a) examine possible mechanisms that could produce abnormally rapid action potentials for a prolonged period and (b) search for NTs that might be temporarily disabled by this behavior and develop depression. This required a detailed study of ion channels that have a dominant role in resting potentials and action potentials.

References

58. Wade, N. J., & Brozek, J. (2001). *Purkinje's vision: The dawning of neuroscience*. Psychology Press.

59. Golgi, C. (1967). The Neuron Doctrine—Theory and Facts. From Nobel Lectures, Physiology or Medicine 1901–1921.

60. Ramon y Cajal, S. (1967). The structure and connexions of neurons. From Nobel Lectures, Physiology or Medicine 1901–1921.

61. Sherrington, C. S. (1926). *The integrative action of the nervous system.* Yale University Press.

62. Levitan, I. B., & Kaczmarek, L. K. (2015). *The Neuron: Cell and Molecular Biology.* Oxford University Press.

63. Cooper, G. M. (2000). *The cell: A molecular approach.* ASM Press; Sinauer Associates.

64. Raza, M. U., Tufan, T., Wang, Y., Hill, C., & Zhu, M. Y. (2016). DNA damage in major psychiatric diseases. *Neurotoxicity research, 30,* 251–267.

65. Huang, C. Y. M., & Rasband, M. N. (2018). Axon initial segments: structure, function, and disease. *Annals of the New York Academy of Sciences, 1420*(1), 46–61.

66. McCoy, A. N., & Tan, Y. S. (2014). Otto loewi (1873–1961): Dreamer and nobel laureate. *Singapore medical journal, 55*(1), 3.

67. Beckstead, R. M. (1996). The Life Cycle of Neurotransmitters. In *A Survey of Medical Neuroscience* (pp. 32–44). Springer, New York, NY.

68. Wimalasena, K. (2011). Vesicular monoamine transporters: Structure-function, pharmacology, and medicinal chemistry. *Medicinal research reviews, 31*(4), 483–519.

69. Purves D., Augustine G. J., Fitzpatrick D., et al., editors. *Neuroscience. 2nd edition.* Sunderland (MA): Sinauer Associates; 2001. Chapter 7, Neurotransmitter Receptors and Their Effects.

70. Barnett, Mark & Larkman, Philip. (2007). The action potential. *Practical neurology, 7.* 192–7.

CHAPTER 4

Ion Channels

During periods of solitude and relaxation, one might get the impression that brain activity has slowed and very little is going on. This is far from the truth, and the frenetic and continuous movement of ion channels is a good example. There is an astonishing amount of ion channel activity in our brains even when we are asleep. A typical neuron has about 10,000 ion channels scattered throughout its membrane. Ion channel lifetimes range from hours to days, and more than 1 billion are replaced every second. Humans have a team of more than 400 ion channels that orchestrate complex neuronal behavior. It is remarkable that the various channel subtypes take up residence at precise locations that are optimal for neurotransmission. However, things do not always go perfectly, and there is increasing evidence that ion channel mutations and displacements are major features of bipolar disorder.[71,72]

Brain neurons may be thought of as tiny excitable battery cells or capacitors that discharge (or fire) to initiate a neurotransmission event. Each neuron is enclosed by an extremely thin plasma membrane containing a variety of ion channel structures. The lipid bilayer membranes are effective electrical insulators, but ion channels permit electrically charged atoms (ions) to cross the membrane. These channels are intimately involved in the establishment of neuron voltages, firing of brain cells, release of NTs, and the return of neurons to their initial condition after an action potential. Neuron firing and neurotransmission could not occur without coordinated functioning of ion channels. The major ion channels classes are shown in Figure 8.

Ion channels are protein structures that snake in and out of neuronal membranes and provide passageways for ions. Many of them have four subunits composed of complex proteins, but others are single molecules. Sodium-potassium pumps fueled by mitochondrial ATP maintain high K^+ and Na^+ gradients across neuronal membranes.[73] In contrast, leak channels for Na^+, K^+, and Cl^- ions function independently without energy support.[74] Leak channels are always open, while voltage-gated channels are closed except for a fraction of a second after the membrane attains a specific threshold voltage.[75] Receptors are special ion channels that open briefly after interacting with a specific NT.

Major Neuron Ion Channels

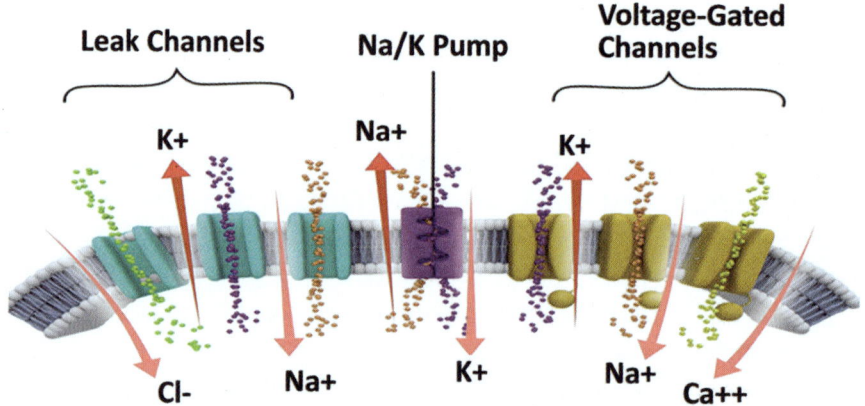

- Na/K Pump: Continous Operation
- Leak Channels: Always Open
- Voltage Gated Channels
  - Usually Closed
  - Open if Threshold Voltage Attained

Figure 8. Major Neuron Ion Channels

I like to compare a neuron's activity to the firing of a gun. In this context, the "gun" is "loaded" by Na/K pumps that produce large K^+ and Na^+ gradients across the membrane. Voltage-gated Na^+ ion channels act as the "trigger" by suddenly opening and reversing membrane polarity. This voltage change causes Ca^{++} ions to rush into the neuron and fire NT "bullets" into the synapse.

Sodium-Potassium Exchange Pump

Healthy brain neurons have high K^+ and low Na^+ levels in their interior cytosol fluid. Large K^+ and Na^+ gradients across neuron membranes are an essential feature of brain function. Danish scientist Jens Skou received the Nobel Prize for his 1957 discovery of the sodium-potassium pump that is responsible for these ion gradients.[76] He detected the presence of membrane proteins that preferentially transport Na^+ ions out of the cell and pump K^+ ions into the cell. Powered by ATP from the mitochondria, these pumps send three Na^+ ions out of the neuron for every two K^+ ions sent inward. At steady state, K^+ concentrations inside the neuron are about 20 times higher than exterior levels, while Na^+ ion concentrations outside the neuron are about nine times that of the interior. The ion concentration gradients enable an electrical field or voltage across the membrane of about -70 mV. By convention, this neuron voltage is considered negative. These pumps work nonstop to maintain the large Na^+ and K^+ gradients across the membrane. Some refer to this as "charging up the membrane battery."

The detailed structure and mechanisms of sodium-potassium pumps are now well known. Unlike mechanical pumps with many parts, they are actually single molecules (Na^+/K^+-ATPase) embedded into neuronal membranes. Like most ion channels, they directly contact both the interior and exterior fluids of a cell. They react with ATP that provides chemical energy to transport ions uphill against large concentration gradients. Reaction with ATP causes three internal Na^+ ions to bind to the ion channel molecule that then twists around to expose the Na^+ ions to the external fluids. After Na^+ ions are released, two external K^+ ions bind to the molecule that twists back to the original shape and deposits them into the interior. The Na/K pump is a workhorse that continuously imports K^+ ions and exports Na^+ ions to produce an excitable neuron capable of ejecting NTs into a synapse. Every time a neuron fires, Na^+ ions rush into the cell, and K^+ ions are lost. The Na/K pumps quickly and efficiently restore the interior fluid to its original ionic composition. In the past few years, we have learned that Na/K pumps also perform complex signaling and have a special role in regulating cerebellum motor activities. In collaboration with inhibitory Purkinje neurons, they enable smooth, well-controlled movements. Alcohol weakens Na/K pump function, which may cause classic symptoms of drunkenness (inebriation).[77] In addition, a mutation in the Na/K pump enzyme can cause a serious form of

Parkinson's disease.[78] Humans have four different Na/K pump sub-types (called isoforms) with unique properties and expression patterns. As neuroscience advances, the complexity and beautiful coordination of ion channels are becoming better defined.

Leak Channels

Some ion channels are constantly open, allowing ions to leak across the membrane at a low rate.[78] Others are voltage-gated and are closed except for a brief period during cell firing. Leak channels determine the resting potential (voltage) of a neuron prior to firing.[79] Their contribution to resting voltage depends on two factors: (a) ion concentration gradients across the neuron membrane and (b) the rate of ion flow (ion permeability) through the channels. Na^+, K^+, and Cl^- represent the major leak channels in a neuron. Outward flow of K^+ ions and influx of Cl^- ions tend to produce a calming negative membrane voltage, whereas inward Na^+ and Ca^{++} ions can sharply increase neuronal excitability. As described later in this chapter and Appendix B, a neuron's resting voltage is dominated by potassium due to the relatively high population of K^+ leak channels.

Voltage-Gated Sodium Channels

These special channels are completely closed when a neuron is at rest. When neuron voltage reaches threshold, they open for about a millisecond and the inrush of Na^+ ions reverses membrane polarity to trigger a neuron firing event (action potential). Voltage-gated Na^+ channels are found throughout neuronal membranes but are highly concentrated at the AIS and the nodes of Ranvier.[79] These channels consist of a large alpha subunit with 1,800 amino acids attached to a beta subunit. The alpha protein crosses in and out of the membrane 24 times, and the S1-S4 zone in the VGSC contains a simple voltage sensor that continuously determines the neuron's net voltage and initiates neuron firing if threshold voltage is reached. The S4 loop has an array of positively charged arginine proteins that exert an electrostatic force on the neuronal membrane that keeps the ion channel pore closed at rest. At threshold voltage, the alpha structure changes shape to form a pore, resulting in a sudden influx of Na^+ ions that triggers an action potential. After about a millisecond, the membrane voltage changes from negative to positive, and inactivation gates shut off the entry of Na⁺ ions. The smaller beta subunits regulate channel gating, modulate expression, and attach to various axon proteins.

Not all voltage-gated sodium channels are the same. In humans, 23 genes are dedicated to voltage-gated Na⁺ channels and produce a family of nine alpha subtypes labeled $Na_v1.1$ to $Na_v1.9$, which perform specialized functions in different locations. $Na_v1.1$ is encoded by the SCN1A gene, and it has a prominent role in regulating the firing rate of GABA neurons. Mutations in this gene are known to cause neuronal hyperactivity and epilepsy. In another example, $Na_v1.6$ ion channels enable rapid-burst neuronal firing. Other Na_v family members have roles in ion channel positioning, pain sensation, repair of damaged neurons, and immune function.

The high population of voltage-gated Na⁺ channels at the neuron's AIS control center sums the voltage changes from incoming neurotransmissions. Action potential initiation is dominated by $Na_v1.6$ ions located at distal (relatively far from the soma) AIS locations. If voltage reaches threshold, a multitude of $Na_v1.6$ channels open to trigger a neuron firing event. High concentrations of $Na_v1.6$ channels at the nodes of Ranvier act as power boosters for the voltage wave traveling down the axon. A considerable amount of research is aimed at the molecular mechanisms that guide members of the Na_v family to specific locations. At later stages of neuronal firing, $Na_v1.2$ ion channels open to send a voltage pulse into the soma and dendrites to release NTs still docked at receptors (to erase the memory of the previous action potential). We recently learned that neurons respond to neuronal hyperactivity by placing Na_v channels farther from the soma to reduce neuron activity.

Voltage-Gated Potassium Channels

Voltage-gated K⁺ channels are transmembrane channels that are closed except during neuron firing events. They play a crucial role in restoring the depolarized cell to its resting state.[80] These channels open about a millisecond after a neuron fires. The resulting outward flow of K⁺ ions quickly restores the resting potential in preparation for the next firing event. This enables some neurons to fire up to 200 times per second. Like most voltage-gated channels, they have high concentrations of positively charged arginine residues that alter channel shape at increased voltages to open a pore. Some of the K⁺ ions departing the neuron are taken up by astrocyte glial cells to avoid excessive K$^+$ build-up in the extracellular space. Impaired clearance of K$^+$ ions outside the neuronal membrane is associated with neuronal hyperactivity.

A multitude of voltage-gated K$^+$ channel subtypes perform specific functions and operate in different brain areas. There are 40 different alpha subunits and 12 beta subunits that provide versatility in function. The major subtypes include outward-rectifying, inward-rectifying, slowly activating, rapidly inactivating, and delayed-rectifying channels. It's not surprising that 50% of the genome's ion-channel genes manage the complex functions of potassium ion channels.

Voltage-Gated Calcium Channels

Calcium pumps powered by ATP remove almost all Ca^{++} ions from the interior of brain neurons.[81] At rest, the concentration of Ca^{++} ions outside the cell is about 10,000 times that of the interior. Voltage-gated Ca^{++} channels are expressed in high numbers at the axon terminus where NTs are stored in vesicles. When a neuron fires, the voltage pulse reaches the axon terminus and briefly opens Ca^{++} channels, suddenly increasing interior Ca^{++} concentrations by a factor of 200. This temporary Ca^{++} influx produces two effects essential to brain function: (1) the Ca^{++} ions cause vesicles to fuse to the membrane and launch NTs into the synapse, and (2) they open calcium-activated K$^+$ channels to quickly re-establish the resting voltage in preparation for the next neuron firing event. The voltage-gated K$^+$ channels close after about a millisecond, completing the neuron's return to its resting voltage.

Calcium-Activated Potassium Channels

These potassium channels are closed except during action potentials when Ca^{++} ions enter the neuron to drive NTs into the synapse.[82] The resulting K$^+$ ion outflow speeds neuron recovery (repolarization) by quickly restoring membrane potential to its original voltage. This allows certain neurons to fire very rapidly, which may be important in brain plasticity, memory formation, and other brain functions.

Chloride Channels

Potassium/Chloride pumps continuously maintain interior Cl$^-$ concentrations at a very low level.[83] At equilibrium, the concentration of extracellular Cl$^-$ is about 20 times that of the cell's interior. Chloride leak channels in the axon and soma are always open and allow continuous inward transport of Cl⁻ ions down the concentration gradient. However, the Cl⁻ ion flow rate (ion permeability) from leak channels is very small compared to that of potassium ions and has a negligible influence on resting voltage. However, chloride channels at GABA receptors contribute to the brain's calming capability. When GABA receptors are activated, the inward flow of negatively charged Cl⁻ ions inhibits neuron firing by moving membrane potential farther from threshold.

Resting Voltage and the Dominance of Potassium

Resting voltages are of special interest in bipolar disorder since reduced levels are associated with neuronal hyperactivity that could produce mania. In this study, we examined various epigenetic and environmental conditions that could cause rest potentials to move closer to the threshold for firing. A neuron's voltage (or potential) at any time depends on the combination of Na^+, K^+, and Cl^- gradients across the membrane. As mentioned previously, resting voltage depends on two factors: (a) the ion concentration gradients across the membrane, and (b) the permeability through the different leak channels. Calcium ion channels do not contribute to this voltage since they are closed (zero permeability) when the neuron is at rest. A neuron's resting voltage may be calculated using the Goldman equation, an extension of the famous Nernst equation (described in Appendix A). The Goldman equation combines the impacts of the individual Na^+, K^+, and Cl^- concentration gradients and their flow rates. In 1949, Hodgkin and Katz[25] discovered that the permeability of potassium ions in neuronal membranes far exceeds that of other ions due to the relatively high population of K^+ leak channels.[84] At rest, flow rates through the sparse Na^+ and Cl^- channels are relatively low and have minimal effect on resting voltage. As a result, neuron resting voltage is roughly proportional to the logarithm of the K^+ concentration gradient, in accordance with the Nernst equation.[85] The resting neuron voltage of about -70 mV is dominated by the K^+ ion gradient across the membrane. If the K^+ concentration gradient was to diminish, membrane resting voltage would move closer to the firing threshold causing the neuron to become more hyperactive. A neuron will fire only if NT "messages" from other neurons bring membrane voltage to the firing threshold.

Ion Channels and Bipolar Disorder

For many years, misbehaving ion channels have been considered a major factor in bipolar disorder switching between neuronal hyperactivity and hypoactivity, and numerous studies have confirmed this belief.[71,72] This inspired my search for specific ion-channel defects that could explain mania onset and increasing severity. A leading suspect was potassium buildup outside neurons that could cause progressive neuronal hyperactivity. I soon learned that astrocyte glial cells pack around axons and assist in removing excess K^+ ions during action potentials. Chapter 5 summarizes the many mechanisms and functions of glial cells that may have a key role in the etiology of bipolar disorder.

References

71. Judy, J. T., Seifuddin, F., Pirooznia, M., Mahon, P. B., Bipolar Genome Study Consortium, Jancic, D., ... & Zandi, P. P. (2013). Converging evidence for epistasis between ANK3 and potassium channel gene KCNQ2 in bipolar disorder. *Frontiers in genetics*, *4*, 87.

72. Harrison, P. J., Hall, N., Mould, A., Al-Juffali, N., & Tunbridge, E. M. (2021). Cellular calcium in bipolar disorder: systematic review and meta-analysis. *Molecular psychiatry*, *26*(8), 4106–4116.

73. Clausen, M. V., Hilbers, F., & Poulsen, H. (2017). The structure and function of the Na, K-ATPase isoforms in health and disease. *Frontiers in physiology*, *8*, 371.

74. Ren, D. (2011). Sodium leak channels in neuronal excitability and rhythmic behaviors. *Neuron*, *72*(6), 899–911.

75. Yu, F. H., & Catterall, W. A. (2003). Overview of the voltage-gated sodium channel family. *Genome biology*, *4*, 1–7.

76. Skou, J. C. (1965). Enzymatic basis for active transport of Na+ and K+ across cell membrane. *Physiological reviews*, *45*(3), 596–618.

77. Zamai, T. N., Titova, N. M., Zamai, A. S., Usol'tseva, O. S., Yulenkova, O. V., & Shumkova, D. A. (2002). Effect of alcoholic intoxication on water content and activity of Na, K-ATPase and Ca-ATPase in rat brain. *Bulletin of Experimental Biology and Medicine*, *134*(6), 541–543.

78. Zhang, X., Lee, W., & Bian, J. S. (2022). Recent advances in the study of Na+/K+-ATPase in neurodegenerative diseases. *Cells, 11*(24), 4075.

79. Alberts B, Johnson A, Lewis J, et al. *Molecular Biology of the Cell. 4th edition.* New York: Garland Science; 2002.

80. Blatz, A. L., & Magleby, K. L. (1987). Calcium-activated potassium channels. *Trends in Neurosciences, 10*(11), 463–467.

81. Brini, M., & Carafoli, E. (2009). Calcium pumps in health and disease. *Physiological reviews, 89*(4), 1341–1378.

82. Latorre, R., Oberhauser, A., Labarca, P., & Alvarez, O. (1989). Varieties of calcium-activated potassium channels. *Annual review of physiology, 51*(1), 385–399.

83. Alvarez-Leefmans, F. J., & Delpire, E. (Eds.). (2009). *Physiology and pathology of chloride transporters and channels in the nervous system: from molecules to diseases.* Academic Press.

84. Huxley, A. F. (2002). Hodgkin and the action potential 1935–1952. *The Journal of physiology, 538*(Pt 1), 2.

85. Feiner, A. S., & McEvoy, A. J. (1994). The nernst equation. *Journal of chemical education, 71*(6), 493.

CHAPTER 5

Glial Cells

In 1836 Germany, 20-year-old Robert Remak's doctoral thesis reported his observation that brain axons were surrounded by very different cells he called ensheathments.[86] Twenty years later, the eminent German scientist Rudolf Virchow published a classic paper stating that brain cells could be divided into two distinct groups: (a) neurons and (b) more numerous cells, which he called "neuroglia" (or "nerve glue"). Remak later complained that Virchow was taking credit for his discovery that he hadn't yet published. For the next 125 years, brain research focused on neurons, with very little attention given to glia, which were considered to be merely physical support for the fragile neurons. This belief was shattered in the 1980s by a remarkable chain of events triggered by scientific studies of Albert Einstein's brain.[87]

Einstein's Last Gift to the World

Albert Einstein died in 1955 at the age of 76 in Princeton, New Jersey. During the autopsy, pathologist Thomas Harvey secretly (and illegally) removed Einstein's brain and preserved it in formaldehyde before the body was cremated. Harvey spent three months preparing and cataloging thousands of slides containing thin slices of Einstein's brain. For several years, Harvey and several colleagues attempted to find unique brain features that could explain Einstein's extraordinary intelligence, but their efforts failed.[88] In 1978, the existence of Einstein's preserved brain was discovered by an investigative reporter. Einstein's family decided they wouldn't pursue criminal action if Harvey would send the brain specimens to experts for scientific research. Initial studies by Dr. Marian Diamond at the University of California, Berkeley, were disappointing.[89] Einstein's brain was no larger than normal brains, and his neurons were quite ordinary in size and number. However, later studies reported a striking abnormality: parts of Einstein's brain contained twice as many glial cells as the number present in most human brains! It was especially intriguing that the biggest difference was in the parietal cortex, a region where abstract concepts and complex thinking take place. This unexpected result suggested to neuroscientists that glial cells are not just physical support for neurons but also have an active role in brain function.

Subsequent studies suggested that the glia/neuron ratio was strongly related to intelligence. For example, the glia/neuron ratio in human brains is 27 times that of rodent brains. The distribution of glial cells is far from uniform, with the highest populations found in the brain's white matter. Brain areas of low neuronal density are assumed to have higher numbers of glial cells. Larger neurons are believed to require extra glial cells to meet their energy and nourishment needs. Most textbooks state that glial cells outnumber neurons by a wide margin, but there is recent experimental evidence that the numbers are approximately equal.[90] This debate will eventually be resolved when researchers divide entire brains into a multitude of thin sections and actually count the numbers of neurons and glia.

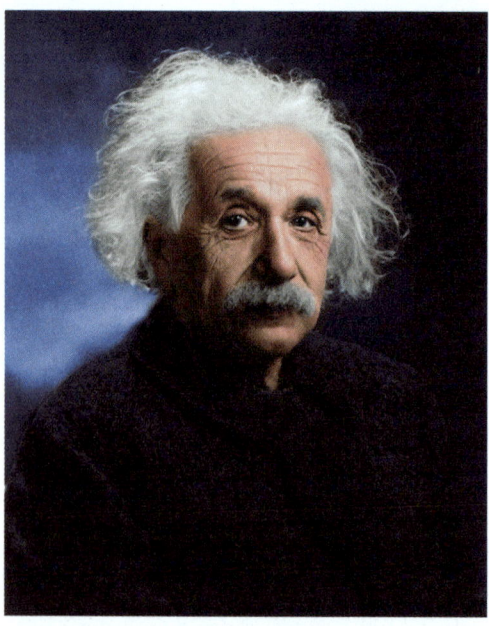

Figure 9. Albert Einstein (1879–1955)

In an ironic twist, recent experimental evidence suggests that the glia/ neuron ratio may not be very significant with respect to intelligence, and this has become an area of controversy and debate.[91] However, all parties agree that glial cells have vast importance in mental health. The studies of Einstein's brain have led to a revolution in brain science that will require rewriting neuroscience textbooks. The "binary" model which depicts neurotransmission as the interaction of a presynaptic and a postsynaptic neuron now must be replaced by a "ternary" model that includes glial cells.[92]

We are now experiencing an explosion in glial cell research, ending a century of neglect.[93,94,95] Researchers have discovered that glial cells have many essential roles in brain function and work in close partnership with neurons. Essential functions of glia include the following:

- In utero production of neurons (neurogenesis)
- Scaffolding for neuronal growth and migration
- Structural support for neurons
- Development of myelin sheaths
- Regulation of nutrient delivery to neurons
- Brain plasticity, including development of new synapses
- Uptake and metabolism of key neurotransmitters
- Potassium ion clearance from outside neuron membranes
- Formation and storage of memory
- Regulation of neuron firing
- Participation in immune function
- Signaling between neurons
- Regulation of the brain's blood supply
- Repair of damaged neurons
- Removal of brain debris

The Birth of the Brain

Glial cells are not only important in neuron functioning, but they are also the original *source* of neurons.[96] During fetal development, specialized radial glial cells develop progenitor stem cells that produce all the brain's neurons and astrocytes. The radial cells span the six cortex layers and provide scaffolding for developing neurons and directions for their migration. During week five of gestation, they generate neurons at an astonishing rate of 250,000 per minute. These special glial cells exclusively produce neurons during early gestation. After most neuron production is complete, the radial stem cells are modified by specific transcription factors to rapidly generate billions of glial cells. Most radial glia disappear after construction of the brain is completed, putting the brakes on neuron production after birth. A few of these progenitor cells remain throughout life and generate new neurons, especially in the dendrite gyrus of the hippocampus and the subventricular zone.

Astrocytes

The human brain contains billions of astrocyte glial cells. They have a star-like appearance with long arms radiating from a central cell body.[97] Like other cells in the body, they have a nucleus containing DNA, mitochondria, Golgi apparatus, and other organelles that are enclosed within a bilayer membrane. Unlike neurons, they are capable of mitosis (cell division), and most glia do not develop action potentials. Astrocytes crowd closely around neuron axons forming an extracellular space about 20 nanometers (nm) wide. Astrocyte cells are in intimate contact with each other and are connected by gap junctions that enable a rapid flow of ions and communication throughout the glial network. Their long star-like arms wrap around blood vessels like bat wings and absorb a constant stream of nutrients for delivery to neurons through the gap junctions. Astrocytes assist in regulation of neuron firing by removing excess K^+ ions from the extracellular space and dumping them into the bloodstream. Waves of Ca^{++} ions spread rapidly throughout the billions of astrocytes to signal neuron firing events. Astrocytes absorb certain neurotransmitters from synapses to help regulate neurotransmission. For example, they take up glutamate from NMDA synapses for conversion to glutamine and transport back into the presynaptic neuron. This NMDA reuptake process appears clumsy and inefficient but plays a key role in memory formation. Researchers recently learned that astrocyte membranes contain receptors that can take up and release neurotransmitters. Some neuroscientists believe that astrocytes form synapses with neurons and are major partners in brain functioning. Funding for astrocyte research has sharply increased in recent years.

The Magic of Myelin

Myelin is a white fatty substance (80% lipids) that collects around axons and acts as an electrical insulator.[98] The myelin sheath is formed by glial cells with a peculiar shape and even stranger name – *oligoden-drocytes*, a Greek expression for "stubby branches." These cells have a round cell body with numerous short arms that wrap tightly around axons. Some researchers compare their shape to that of an octopus. It is quite remarkable that myelin is formed only on axons, separated by precisely located gaps called nodes of Ranvier. Each myelin sheath contains layers of glial membranes, with the interior fluid squeezed out like empty tubes of toothpaste. There is no gap between myelin and axons, rendering the sheath impervious to electrons and metal ions. Myelin (a) provides electrical isolation of axons from other brain cells, (b) enables rapid conduction of action potentials, and (c) provides narrow spaces for nodes of Ranvier and their power-boosting Na$^+$ ion channels. Most myelin is found in the white matter of the brain, with lesser amounts in gray matter. Myelin-related disorders include multiple sclerosis, Guillain-Barre syndrome (GBS), and several others. Myelin is an essential element in efficient neuron firing and neurotransmission. Without myelin, we might have the intelligence of a fruit fly.

Microglia – The Brain's Immune System[99,100]

The brain's isolation behind the BBB deprives it of robust access to the body's immune system that combats infection and disease. The brain instead has its own defense army, a type of glial cell called microglia. Billions of small dynamic microglia are distributed throughout the brain lying in wait to defend against infection or injury. Like soldiers in camouflage, they change shape when alerted to infection or injury and rush with remarkable speed to the problem area to devour a virus or bacterium or assist in repair of damaged neurons. Microglia have an impressive array of sensors that detect danger and are equipped with healing proteins that repair neurons. They also have a role in rewiring neuron circuits and learning.

Microglia possess impressive ability to protect the brain, but they can be very harmful if they release excessive amounts of inflammatory cytokines or free radicals. There is accumulating evidence that microglia dysregulation contributes to Alzheimer's disease, amyotrophic lateral sclerosis (ALS), Parkinson's disease, OCD, Tourette syndrome (TS), and pediatric autoimmune neuropsychiatric disorders associated with streptococcal infections (PANDAS).

Until recently, it was believed that the body's lymphatic system did not reach the brain and that microglia represented the brain's only significant immune capability. However, in 2015, special gadolinium-staining techniques revealed that tiny lymph vessels enter the brain through the closely packed pia mater and other layers of the meninges.[101,102] This surprising discovery indicates that lymph participates in the brain's immunity and assists in the removal of fluid and large molecules. The relative contributions of lymph and microglia to the brain's immune capability are presently unknown.

References

86. Kettenmann, H. and Ransom, B.R. (2005) *Neuroglia*. Oxford University Press, Oxford.

87. Fields, R. D. (2009). *The other brain: From dementia to schizophrenia, how new discoveries about the brain are revolutionizing medicine and science*. Simon and Schuster.

88. Witelson, S. F., Kigar, D. L., & Harvey, T. (1999). The exceptional brain of Albert Einstein. *The Lancet, 353*(9170), 2149–2153.

89. Diamond, M. C., Scheibel, A. B., Murphy Jr, G. M., & Harvey, T. (1985). On the brain of a scientist: Albert Einstein. *Experimental neurology, 88*(1), 198–204.

90. Verkhratsky, A., & Butt, A. M. (2018). The history of the decline and fall of the glial numbers legend. *Neuroglia, 1*(1), 188–192.

91. Songthawornpong, N., Teasdale, T. W., Olesen, M. V., & Pakkenberg, B. (2021). Is there a correlation between the number of brain cells and IQ?. *Cerebral Cortex, 31*(1), 650–657.

92. Purves D., Augustine G. J., Fitzpatrick D., et al., editors. *Neuroscience. 2nd edition*. Sunderland (MA): Sinauer Associates; 2001. Chapter 1, Neuroglial Cells.

93. Noctor, S. C., Flint, A. C., Weissman, T. A., Dammerman, R. S., & Kriegstein, A. R. (2001). Neurons derived from radial glial cells establish radial units in neocortex. *Nature, 409*(6821), 714–720.

94. Hanani, M., & Verkhratsky, A. (2021). Satellite glial cells and astrocytes, a comparative review. *Neurochemical research, 46*(10), 2525–2537.

95. Wartchow, K. M., Scaini, G., & Quevedo, J. (2023). Glial-neuronal interaction in synapses: A possible mechanism of the pathophysiology of bipolar disorder. *Neuroinflammation, Gut-Brain Axis and Immunity in Neuropsychiatric Disorders*, 191–208.

96.   Liu, S. H., Du, Y., Chen, L., & Cheng, Y. (2022). Glial cell
       abnormalities in major psychiatric diseases: A systematic review
       of postmortem brain studies. *Molecular neurobiology, 59*(3),
       1665–1692.
97.   Vasile, F., Dossi, E., & Rouach, N. (2017). Human astrocytes:
       structure and functions in the healthy brain. *Brain structure &
       function, 222*(5), 2017–2029.
98.   Morell P., Quarles R. H. The Myelin Sheath. In: Siegel GJ, Agranoff
       BW, Albers RW, et al., editors. *Basic Neurochemistry: Molecular,
       Cellular and Medical Aspects. 6th edition.* Philadelphia: Lippincott-
       Raven; 1999.
99.   Li, Q., & Barres, B. A. (2018). Microglia and macrophages in brain
       homeostasis and disease. *Nature Reviews Immunology, 18*(4),
       225–242.
100.   Hanisch, U. K., & Kettenmann, H. (2007). Microglia: active sensor
       and versatile effector cells in the normal and pathologic brain. *Nature
       neuroscience, 10*(11), 1387–1394.
101.   Louveau, A., Smirnov, I., Keyes, T. J., Eccles, J. D., Rouhani, S. J.,
       Peske, J. D., ... & Kipnis, J. (2015). Structural and functional features
       of central nervous system lymphatic vessels. *Nature, 523*(7560),
       337–341.
102.   Bucchieri, F., Farina, F., Zummo, G., & Cappello, F. (2015).
       Lymphatic vessels of the dura mater: a new discovery?. *Journal of
       Anatomy, 227*(5), 702.

CHAPTER 6

DNA – The Molecule of Life

A Brief History of DNA

In 1869, Swiss chemist Johann Friedrich Miescher found a strange phosphorus-containing substance he called "nuclein" while studying white blood cells.[103] Miescher had no idea that he had just discovered the most important molecule in human biochemistry. Twelve years later, German biochemist Albrecht Kossel determined the substance was a nucleic acid and named it "deoxyribonucleic acid" (DNA).[104] Despite primitive equipment, Kossel also identified DNA's four building block sub-molecules (adenine, cytosine, guanine, and thymine) and received the Nobel Prize for this brilliant work. This led to a series of remarkable discoveries over the next 25 years.[105] German scientists Schleiden, Virchow, and Bütschli identified and studied important segments of DNA now known as chromosomes. Walter Flemming discovered the mechanism of mitosis and the key role of chromosomes. In 1902, Walter Sutton and Theodor Boveri independently developed the chromosome theory of inheritance. Theophilus Painter famously published his finding of 24 chromosome pairs in human DNA in 1923, an error that persisted until 1956 when J. H. Tjio proved the correct number was 23 chromosome pairs.[106]

The early work of Gregor Mendel proved that life forms transmit characteristic traits during reproduction. However, there were many years of debate and controversy before DNA was conclusively proven in 1943 to be the bearer of inherited traits.[107] This launched a legendary scientific race to determine the structure and chemistry of DNA, now clearly the most important molecule in biochemistry. The early leader in the race was Nobel laureate Linus Pauling, who discovered DNA's helix structure.[108] James Watson learned that Pauling's triple helix model was incorrect, after viewing an X-ray crystallography DNA image from Rosalind Franklin's lab during a visit to London in 1952. One of Franklin's colleagues showed the image to Watson (without her knowledge) before she could publish the discovery herself. Franklin's famous Image 51 decisively revealed DNA's double helix structure.[109] In 1953, James Watson and Francis Crick published a DNA model that correctly describes a double helix molecule that twists to form a ladder-like structure, with paired cytosine-guanine and adenine-thymine bases forming the rungs.[110] Many believe the discovery of DNA's structure and chemical composition to be the most important scientific discovery in the history of the world.

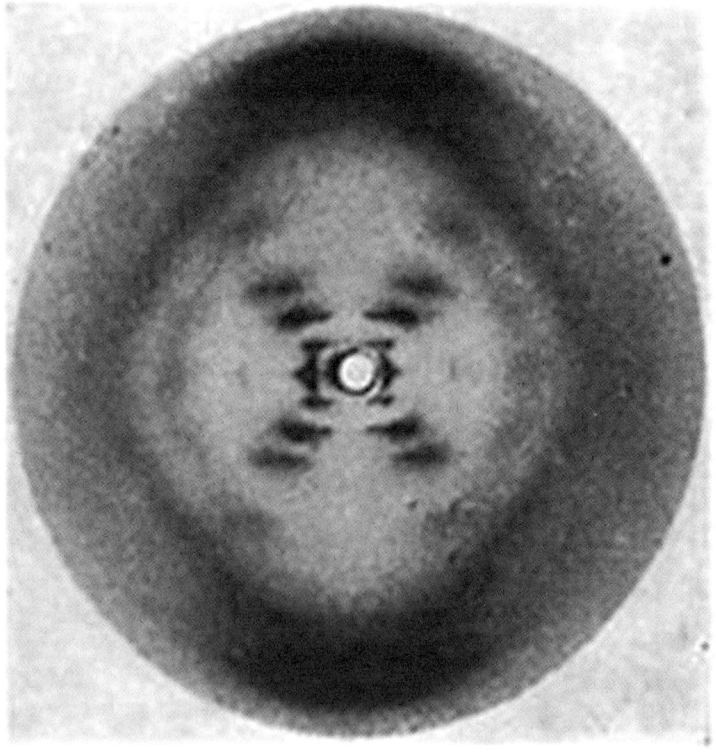

Figure 10. X-Ray Diffraction Image of DNA by
Gosling and Franklin (Image 51)

An afternoon with Linus Pauling: On the occasion of Dr. Pauling's 90th birthday celebration in Chicago, I spent several hours alone with the great scientist and enjoyed a lively discussion of biochemistry and physics. I was excited to learn the world's only winner of two individual Nobel Prizes had been following my research. My enthusiasm was dampened when his first comment was that I was making a big mistake—spending too much time studying the abnormal biochemistry of violent criminals and mental patients, with not nearly enough effort establishing the biochemistry of normal behavior. Of course, he was correct, and I took this advice in my future research.

Pauling didn't want to talk about his Nobel successes but spoke at length about losing the DNA race to Watson and Crick. He blamed his mistaken triple helix model on lab chemistry errors. He also regretted cancelling a visit to Rosalind Franklin's lab the same week as the famous Watson visit to London. His visa to Great Britain was delayed due to pressure from Senator Joseph McCarthy who thought he might have communist leanings.

As we parted, Pauling expressed disappointment at having to reduce his daily vitamin C intake from 20 grams to 18 grams due to digestive problems. He felt the high-dose antioxidant had contributed to his excellent health and mental sharpness. At the evening's dinner dance birthday celebration, Dr. Pauling impressed everyone with his physical vigor and inspiring lecture.

Scientists have learned that all forms of life on earth have DNA with the same building-block nucleotide molecules (adenine, cytosine, guanine, thymine). This includes plants, insects, animals, and humans. All living things, including tiny single-cell amoebae, contain large complex DNA molecules with thousands of base pairs. Even a banana has about 50% of the genes found in humans. DNA is a self-replicating carrier of all genetic information. It contains the instructions needed for organisms to develop, grow, survive, and reproduce.

DNA life forms were once believed unique in the universe since they appear to violate the second law of thermodynamics that specifies that entropy (the degree of randomness) always increases. For example, if you place 50 black jelly beans on top of 50 white jelly beans in a container and shake the container, they will gradually become evenly distributed. This property (sometimes called chaos) applies throughout the universe. Nevertheless, there are many processes in which a living entity's entropy can decline. For example, consumed nutrients do not travel randomly to cells but are distributed in an organized manner resulting in an entropy loss. However, thermodynamic laws involve "closed systems" and aren't violated if we consider life forms together with their surrounding environment. Living entities perform work (a physics concept involving energy transfer) that increases entropy in the environment, resulting in a net entropy gain.

Our vastly improved knowledge of DNA has caused consternation regarding the origin of life on earth. We know that DNA did not exist on Earth 4.5 billion years ago when the Earth was molten, and we also know that life forms did exist 3.8 billion years ago. The question is this: *How* did the first DNA molecule appear on Earth during the intervening 700 million years?[111] An early theory involved a fortuitous combination of molecules aggregating over millions of years in an aqueous environment with lightning or cosmic radiation triggering the first elementary life form (perhaps a single-cell amoeba). However, we have learned even the simplest living entity has very long DNA molecules with extraordinary complexity, and scientists are struggling to develop plausible explanations for natural development or evolution of the first DNA molecule. Recent years have seen increased interest in theories involving meteors that may have brought DNA from outer space. Numerous meteorites have contained crucial components of DNA and RNA, which suggests extraterrestrial origins.[112] A respected RNA world theory assumes that DNA developed from RNA (a less complex molecule), and hundreds of scientists are now seeking a plausible evolutionary model for the origin of RNA.[113] In addition, a growing number of philosophers and religious leaders refer to DNA as the "God molecule" that arrived by metaphysical means.[114] In any case, our huge DNA "life molecules" are quite unique and hold many secrets regarding human existence, including the specific causes and mechanisms of disease conditions. We have only just begun to understand the extraordinary complexities of gene expression, epigenetic variations, and deteriorating DNA integrity that are central to most physical and mental disorders.

During the 70 years since Watson and Crick's discovery, scientists have sequenced the entire human genome, identifying approximately 20,000 genes that code for expressed proteins, and learned how DNA orchestrates a multitude of complex processes essential to life. This book does not attempt a comprehensive description of

DNA and its many properties and functions. Instead, it concentrates on aspects of DNA that have greatest relevance to bipolar disorder.

DNA Nourishment of the Brain and Body

Each person has trillions of DNA molecules that determine eye color, sex, and other inborn characteristics. However, DNA also acts as a workhorse that supervises daily production of special proteins needed by cells, including neurons and glia.[115] We cannot exist for a minute without these genetically expressed proteins. It is becoming clear that bipolar disorder and other late-onset maladies may develop if this cell nourishment is altered or disrupted as we age. Although microscopic in appearance, human DNA strands contain about three billion nucleotide base pairs in the double helix array. If a person's DNA strands were stretched out and attached end-to-end, the total length would exceed 300 times the distance to the sun, which may help us comprehend how DNA contains its extraordinary amount of information. Our 20,000+ coding genes contain blueprints for making vital expressed proteins. Once gestation and early development have been completed, every gene has a single job – to enable production of one or more proteins that might be an enzyme, ion channel, transcription factor, or other important molecule.

DNA's four nucleotide bases: adenine (A), guanine (G), cytosine (C), and thymine (T) provide the unique codes for specifying the amino acid sequence for an expressed protein. Each triplet of three consecutive bases is a codon that identifies one of the 20 amino acid building blocks. There are 64 possible triplet combinations of the bases (A, G, C, T), but only 20 amino acid components in expressed proteins; so, many of the amino acids have more than one triplet code. For example, arginine has four codons (CGT, CGC, CGA, or CGG) that are different aliases for the same amino acid. Two of the 64 codons are start and stop codons, respectively. Depending on the gene, an expressed protein may be quite small and linear or composed of more than 25,000 amino acids that can develop into a complex shape. Each gene's array begins with the start codon, followed by codons that specify the linear protein's amino acid sequence, ending at the stop codon. Aided by RNA polymerase (RNAP) and transcription factors, a gene's amino acid sequence is copied onto special molecules called mRNA that deliver these specifications to ribosomes for protein production. This copying process is known as transcription.

Most sets of gene instructions for expressed proteins are far from perfect and contain mutations called SNPs in which one nucleotide base is out of place. Inherited SNPs present at conception are called germline SNPs, and those that develop during life are termed somatic SNPs. Most SNPs have little or no effect on a protein's function, but others can cause considerable mischief. For example, a C677t SNP mutation in the methylenetetrahydrofolate reductase (MTHFR) gene can reduce enzymatic activity by about two-thirds, resulting in a methylation disorder.[116] In another example, apolipoprotein E (APOE) gene mutations in which cysteine residues are replaced by arginine result in APOE-3 or APOE-4 and cause a higher risk for Alzheimer's disease.[117] Most humans have more than 4 million SNP mutations in their DNA, which suggests we all could be considered mutants. Our inborn (germline) SNP mutations help define our personality, abilities, and vulnerability to diseases. Thousands of expressed proteins have a significant impact on mental health. Examples include (a) ion channel proteins that regulate neuron firing, (b) enzymes that enable synthesis of neurotransmitters, and (c) SERT transporter proteins required for serotonin reuptake. Many birth defects and developmental disorders are caused by germline mutations that alter the structure and biochemical properties of expressed proteins. Inborn mutations can also predispose to bipolar disorder and other late-onset maladies that develop after years of relentless DNA damage. In genetics, the term *gene mutation* is often replaced by the more general term *gene variant*.

In addition to SNPs, there are several other mutation types that can change the configuration and function of expressed proteins. For example, our DNA contains many sites where one or more codons were deleted, and other locations where extraneous codons were inserted. Some mutations associated with bipolar risk involve copy number variations (CNVs) in which there may be more than one copy of a gene along a DNA strand.[118] Some SNPs and other variants may actually represent improvements if an altered protein has advantages in a particular environment due to natural selection. For example, Scandinavians tend to have fair skin and blue eyes, compared to people in other parts of the world, due to reduced exposure to sunlight. We humans share about 99.9% of the same DNA. For each person, it's the 0.1% (one part in a thousand) that makes us different.

The Genetic Restaurant

Humans have about 200 major cell types, and each requires a unique combination of expressed proteins for proper functioning.[119] Each cell type may be thought of as a separate universe in which unique protein expression rates are established during gestation by epigenetic regulating factors. Each cell type enjoys the equivalent of a "genetic restaurant" with a menu of thousands of nutrient proteins that may be selected or avoided. In addition, a protein's expression rate ("portion size") may be quite different for each cell type. To complicate matters, most genes produce more than one protein variant by a mechanism called alternative splicing, in which mRNA may skip codons or incorporate introns (non-coding DNA sequences between coding regions) while transcribing DNA segments.[120] This enables a menu of more than 80,000 proteins available to each cell type. Selection from the menu is partially accomplished by in utero placement of methyl bookmarks on DNA that can reduce or eliminate expression of individual proteins. In addition, protein production rates are fine-tuned by histone reactions, transcription factors, microRNA (miRNA), and other molecules that may or may not be active in a specific cell type.[121] It's quite remarkable that an acceptable combination of expressed nutrients usually is delivered to each of the different cell types and tissues at birth. In a healthy cell, necessary proteins are supplied at the proper rate and unwanted proteins are avoided.

The Miracle of DNA Repair

Most people don't realize that their trillions of precious DNA molecules are under constant severe assault and endure quite shocking damage every day. Our microscopic and fragile DNA molecules have been attacked by cosmic radiation, toxic chemicals, and other insults from the day we were born.[122] Each strand of DNA is ripped apart or chemically altered more than 10,000 times daily. This problem cannot be avoided even in a perfect environment since essential metabolic processes in the body generate free radicals that can damage DNA.

A most remarkable aspect of human existence is DNA repair. The 2015 Nobel Prize in Chemistry was awarded to Tomas Lindahl, Paul L. Modrich, and Aziz Sancar for discovering the complex DNA repair mechanisms that quickly (and astonishingly) restore damaged DNA to its original condition despite single-strand breaks, double-strand breaks, unwanted chemical reactions, and misplaced

amino acids.[123,124,125,126] It's as though each microscopic DNA molecule has a thousand tiny repairmen constantly on the job. DNA repair
maintains proper cell nourishment from expressed proteins, enables
accurate copying during cell division, and combats senescence (the
cell remains but stops functioning), apoptosis (cell death), and cancer.
The repair mechanisms are highly efficient, but not perfect, since the
hundreds of genes that enable DNA repair may have SNP mutations
or experience epigenetic impairments that slowly and gradually accumulate with time. RNA molecules in our cells are similarly attacked
by cosmic radiation, oxidative stress, and chemical agents, which can
cause severe damage to RNA. Very recently, scientists have discovered repair mechanisms that reverse RNA damage.

Despite very impressive repair capabilities, the integrity and effectiveness of our DNA and RNA inevitably deteriorate with time. For
example, mitosis does not produce perfect daughter cells, and typical cells no longer function effectively after 40–60 cell divisions (the
"Hayflick limit"). Declining DNA integrity is the basic reason why we
age and is a major factor in the onset of most human illnesses, including bipolar disorder. Several research groups have reported unusual-
ly-high incidence of single-strand breaks, double-strand breaks, and
chemical adducts in the DNA and RNA of bipolar patients.[127] Although
a major increase in DNA damage at the time of onset has not yet
been proven, I believe that bipolar disorder usually develops due to
loss of DNA integrity and that genetic weakness in DNA repair may
be an important predisposing factor.

DNA repair involves several highly complex processes including
direct reversal, base excision repair (BER), nucleotide excision repair,
mismatch repair, double-strand breaks, homologous recombination,
and non-homologous end joining (NHEJ). Appendix B provides a
detailed summary of these major repair processes that keep us alive
every second of our existence.

Epigenetics and Bipolar Disorder

It's important to understand the relationship between genetics and
epigenetics. At birth, genetics determines the amino acid sequence
of an expressed protein, while epigenetics determines its unique
production rate in each cell type.[128] In other words, genetics defines
the composition of an expressed protein, which may have inborn
SNPs or other mutations, while epigenetics determines how much is

produced in each part of the body. Epigenetics also refers to changes in molecular composition and local expression rates due to loss of DNA integrity with time. It is becoming clear that bipolar disorder risk may involve a combination of (a) inborn predisposing genetic mutations and (b) specific epigenetic impairments in protein quality and expression rates that develop with advancing age.

References

103. Dahm, R. (2005). Friedrich Miescher and the discovery of DNA. *Developmental biology, 278*(2), 274–288.
104. Jones, M. E. (1953). Albrecht Kossel, a biographical sketch. *The Yale journal of biology and medicine, 26*(1), 80.
105. O'Connor, C., & Miko, I. (2008). Developing the chromosome theory. *Nature education, 1*(1), 44.
106. Harper, P. S. (2006). The discovery of the human chromosome number in Lund, 1955–1956. *Human Genetics, 119*, 226–232.
107. Deichmann, U. (2004). Early responses to Avery et al.'s paper on DNA as hereditary material. *Historical studies in the physical and biological sciences, 34*(2), 207–232.
108. Pauling, L., & Corey, R. B. (1953). A proposed structure for the nucleic acids. *Proceedings of the National Academy of Sciences, 39*(2), 84–97.
109. Davies, K. (2020). Rosalind Franklin Scientist: On the centenary of her birth, a look back at the fundamental role of Rosalind Franklin in unravelling the structure of the double helix in 1953.
110. Watson, J. D., & Crick, F. H. (1953). Molecular structure of nucleic acids; a structure for deoxyribose nucleic acid. *Nature, 171*(4356), 737–738.
111. Committee on Planetary Biology, & Chemical Evolution. (1990). *The Search for Life's Origins: Progress and Future Directions in Planetary Biology and Chemical Evolution*. National Academies.
112. Callahan, M. P., Smith, K. E., Cleaves, H. J., Ruzicka, J., Stern, J. C., Glavin, D. P., ... & Dworkin, J. P. (2011). Carbonaceous meteorites contain a wide range of extraterrestrial nucleobases. *Proceedings of the National Academy of Sciences, 108*(34), 13995–13998.
113. Forterre, P. (2003). Origin of DNA and DNA Genomes. *Origins of Life and Evolution of the Biosphere, 33*, 303–304.

114. Weigmann, K. (2004). The code, the text and the language of God: When explaining science and its implications to the lay public, metaphors come in handy. But their indiscriminate use could also easily backfire. *EMBO reports, 5*(2), 116–118.

115. Larson, D. R., Singer, R. H., & Zenklusen, D. (2009). A single molecule view of gene expression. *Trends in cell biology, 19*(11), 630–637.

116. Liew, S. C., & Gupta, E. D. (2015). Methylenetetrahydrofolate reductase (MTHFR) C677T polymorphism: epidemiology, metabolism and the associated diseases. *European journal of medical genetics, 58*(1), 1–10.

117. Serrano-Pozo, A., Das, S., & Hyman, B. T. (2021). APOE and Alzheimer's disease: advances in genetics, pathophysiology, and therapeutic approaches. *The Lancet. Neurology, 20*(1), 68–80.

118. Green, E. K., Rees, E., Walters, J. T. R., Smith, K. G., Forty, L., Grozeva, D., ... & Kirov, G. (2016). Copy number variation in bipolar disorder. *Molecular psychiatry, 21*(1), 89–93.

119. Mostafa, H. K. (2022). Different cells of the human body: categories and morphological characters. *Journal of Microscopy and Ultrastructure, 10*(2), 40–46.

120. Wang, Y., Liu, J., Huang, B. O., Xu, Y. M., Li, J., Huang, L. F., ... & Wang, X. Z. (2015). Mechanism of alternative splicing and its regulation. *Biomedical reports, 3*(2), 152–158.

121. Gibney, E. R., & Nolan, C. M. (2010). Epigenetics and gene expression. *Heredity, 105*(1), 4–13.

122. Martin, L. J. (2008). DNA damage and repair: relevance to mechanisms of neurodegeneration. *Journal of Neuropathology & Experimental Neurology, 67*(5), 377–387.

123. Lindahl, T. (1982). DNA repair enzymes. *Annual review of biochemistry, 51*(1), 61–87.

124. Lindahl, T. (1993). Instability and decay of the primary structure of DNA. *Nature, 362*(6422), 709–715.

125. Sancar, A. (1994). Mechanisms of DNA excision repair. *Science, 266*(5193), 1954–1956.

126. Modrich, P. (2016). Mechanisms in E. coli and human mismatch repair. *Angewandte Chemie (International ed. in English), 55*(30), 8490.

127. Arat Çelik, H. E., Yılmaz, S., Akşahin, İ. C., Kök Kendirlioğlu, B., Çörekli, E., Dal Bekar, N. E., Çelik, Ö. F., Yorguner, N., Targıtay

Öztürk, B., İşlekel, H., Özerdem, A., Akan, P., Ceylan, D., & Tuna, G. (2024). Oxidatively-induced DNA base damage and base excision repair abnormalities in siblings of individuals with bipolar disorder DNA damage and repair in bipolar disorder. *Translational psychiatry*, *14*(1), 207.

128. Felsenfeld, G. (2014). A brief history of epigenetics. *Cold Spring Harbor perspectives in biology*, *6*(1), a018200.

CHAPTER 7

Epigenetics

As described in Chapter 6, genetics determines the chemical composition and structure of our 80,000 expressed proteins, while epigenetic mechanisms regulate expression rates in every part of the body. Each cell type contains identical copies of DNA, but liver, kidneys, brain, and certain other body sites require a unique combination of expressed proteins for optimal health. Epigenetics is essential to human existence. Without variable rates of gene expression, we might be an amorphous blob of identical cells that could not function or even survive. Good health requires a unique combination of expressed proteins tailored to each cell line, and this is accomplished by epigenetics. The three primary epigenetic mechanisms are DNA methylation, histone modification, and non-coding RNA processes.[128,129]

DNA Methylation

Primary control of a gene's expression rate for each cell line is determined in early fetal development by the presence or absence of methyl bookmarks on DNA's CpG islands (clusters of cytosine-guanine repeats connected by phosphorus atoms). In general, a methyl mark tends to slow or prevent gene expression, and the absence of a methyl mark tends to promote expression. At birth, DNA's methyl bookmarks are firmly in place and usually remain throughout life. The positioning of methyl marks may result from genetic inheritance or be altered by in utero environment. DNA bookmarking has a strong impact on intelligence, personality, health, athletic ability, and vulnerability to specific diseases. We are learning that global DNA methylation (the degree to which

DNA is methylated) is associated with neurotransmission variations.[130] I've observed that hypomethylated DNA is generally associated with depressed serotonin activity and elevated glutamate
activity at NMDA receptors, while hypermethylated DNA typically
involves excessive dopamine activity and depressed glutamate
NMDA activity. Interestingly, the lifetime risk of developing bipolar
disorder seems to be relatively unaffected by differences in global
DNA methylation.

Histone Modification

In addition to methyl bookmarking, gene expression rates are fine-
tuned by chemicals that attach to histone proteins which provide a
support structure for DNA.[36,131] As seen in Figure 11, histones are
made up of eight linear proteins that are twisted together like a ball
of yarn. DNA gently wraps around the histone balls due to electrostatic attraction (DNA is a weak acid, and histones are strong
bases). Protein expression rates are modified by the competition
between methyl and acetyl groups at histone tails which protrude
from the ball configuration. Gene expression requires DNA to uncoil
from histones to allow access for large RNA polymerase and transcription factor molecules that constantly swim in the cell nucleus
fluid looking for an exposed gene to express. Methylation increases
a histone's positive charge, whereas acetyl groups make histones
less basic. If acetyl reactions dominate, reduced electrostatic attraction causes DNA to uncoil from the histone and be more available for
expression (Figure 12). If methylation dominates, the DNA/histone
array (called chromatin) is compressed, preventing or slowing gene
expression (Figure 13). Many methyl and acetyl bookmarks on histone tails have low stability, and the majority of early epigenetic therapies involved histone modification that alters the expression rate of
a target gene. For example, methionine or S-adenosyl-L-methionine
(SAMe) supplements can increase serotonin neurotransmission by
reducing expression of SERT reuptake genes. In another example,
folates and other deacetylase inhibitors may increase expression of
cancer prevention genes.

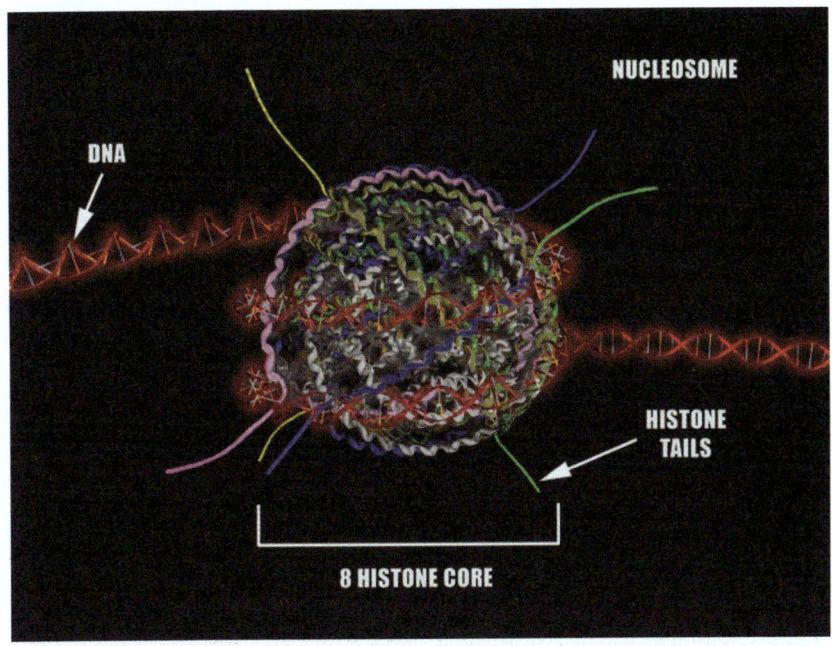

Figure 11. Histone Structure

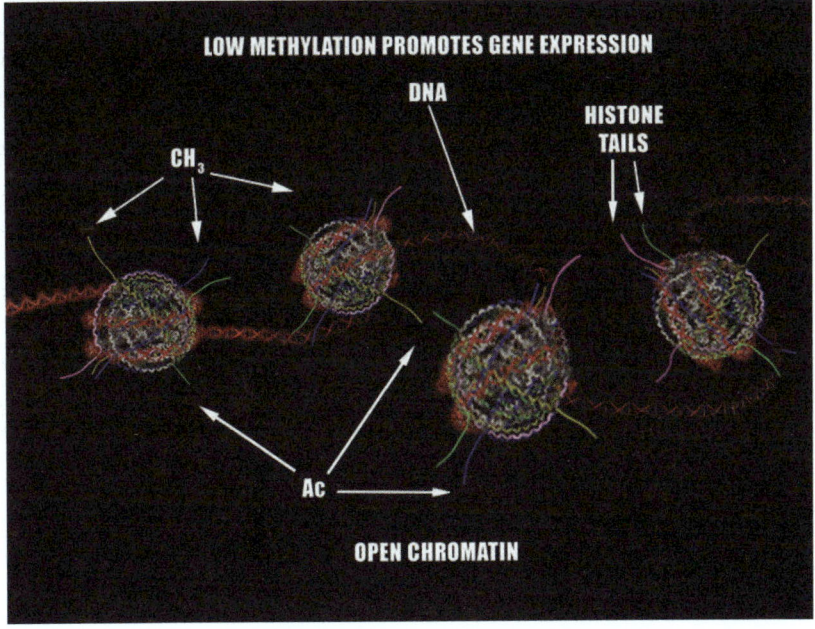

Figure 12. Exposed DNA (Open Chromatin)

RNA Polymerase and Transcription Factors

RNA polymerase (RNAP) is an enzyme that copies a gene's DNA code to form a "loaded mRNA" molecule that delivers the code to ribosomes where proteins are produced. This copying process is called transcription.[132] Transcription factors (TFs) are proteins that assist the transfer of codons from DNA to mRNA and regulate the rate of protein production for each gene. Each TF has a DNA motif that can directly attach to DNA. Many TF proteins have amino acid domains that can sense an exposed gene and guide a RNAP molecule to a gene's promoter zone to start the copying process. There are 1,600 TF genes with somewhat different properties that can tailor protein production to the needs of specific cell types and tissues. Although named for their role in gene transcription, TF proteins also have critical roles during embryonic development.

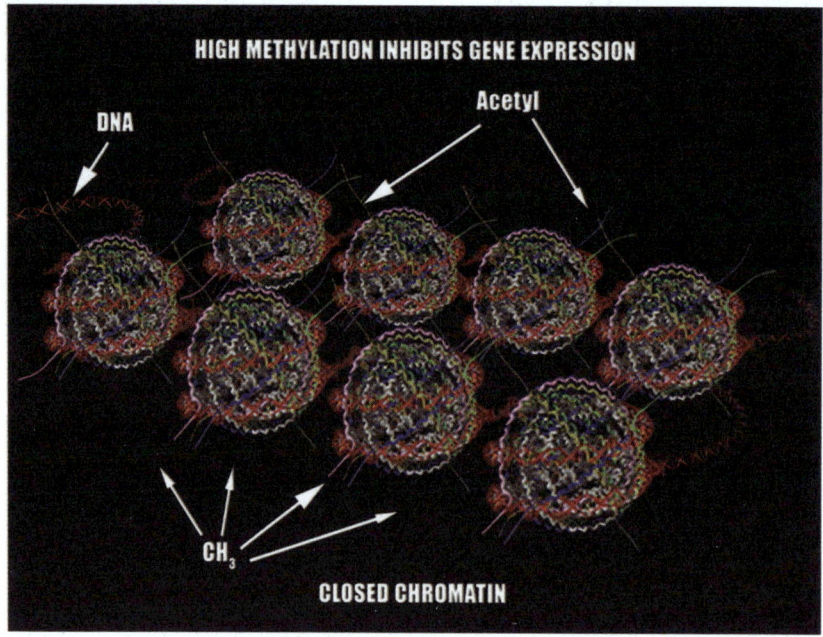

Figure 13. Closed Chromatin

microRNA: The Traffic Cop

After a gene's amino acid sequence has been copied, the loaded mRNA molecule must pass through nuclear membrane pores and travel to a ribosome to produce the target protein. However, many copied DNA sequences are imperfect and are prevented from escaping the cell's nucleus by microRNA (miRNA) molecules. More than 800 genes code for slightly different miRNAs that provide quality control by destroying improperly coded or damaged mRNA. In addition, miRNA molecules can regulate protein production by impacting the rate of loaded mRNAs exiting the nucleus. In addition to miRNA, there are numerous other non-coding RNAs that can either repress or enhance gene expression.[133,134]

Epigenetics enables our identical DNA molecules to provide very different protein combinations tailored to the requirements of each cell type and tissue. This complex process involves thousands of TFs, miRNAs, and other factors that collaborate to meet the needs of individual tissues and cells. Most tissues are developed with amazing precision during the nine months of gestation. During healthy in utero development, thousands of genes collaborate to properly form each tissue. However, this process can be impaired by chemical toxins, radiation, or other environmental insults resulting in subnormal development or malfunctioning of a tissue or organ. The health of a baby depends strongly on their inherited DNA and the epigenetics of protein delivery to each part of the body. Regardless of health status at birth, additional DNA damage gradually accumulates with age in all humans, and resulting impairments in gene expression may be central to bipolar disorder, cancer, and many other late-onset illnesses.

Epigenetic Therapies: Writing, Reading, and Erasing

There is growing evidence that bipolar disorder is associated with damaged genes that gradually accumulate after failed DNA repair. Future epigenetic therapies may effectively cope with this problem. Cancer research has pioneered the development of epigenetic treatments, and this technology is guiding novel treatments for bipolar disorder. The three primary epigenetic anticancer approaches are called *writing, reading,* and *erasing*.[135,136,137] Writing involves modification of gene expression rates through (a) altered placement of methyl bookmarks on DNA or (b) histone modifications that write methyl or acetyl marks at histone tails. Histone modification has dominated early epigenetic applications due to relative instability of methyl, acetyl, or other histone marks that are modified with relative ease. The competition between methyl and acetyl placement at histone tails has a major impact on the degree to which a specific DNA gene is exposed and available for expression. Interestingly, concentrations of methyl and acetyl are far less impactful than methylase, demethylase, acetylase, and deacetylase enzymes and their inhibitors that write the specific mark on a histone tail. Early *writing* therapies have succeeded in enhancing expression of cancer prevention genes.

Second-generation *reading* therapies involve restricting or enhancing access of certain TFs or other transcription modifiers called chromatin *readers* that regulate gene expression rates.[138,139] Damaged TF modifiers containing bromodomain or chromodomain motifs are among the most frequent causes of mutated proteins in human cancers, and drugs that modulate these proteins are under intensive development. Third generation *erasing* therapies are focused on regulating miRNA proteins that prevent imperfect mRNA copies from reaching the cell's protein-production machinery.[140,141] Many miRNAs act to suppress oncogenes and tumors, and there is increasing evidence that aberrant miRNA expressions and signaling pathways are present in important cancers. Researchers have developed miRNA mimics and antagomirs that can normalize gene regulation and signaling. Manipulation of miRNA gene behaviors represents an attractive anticancer approach.

Each of the three cancer treatment approaches (*writing*, *reading*, and *erasing*) has met with considerable success. Many are in FDA trials and others already have achieved FDA approval and are saving lives. In general, reading and erasing therapies enable better specificity (fewer off-target changes) and improved side effect profiles, compared with *writing* therapies. Epigenetic therapies for bipolar disorder are in very early stages of development and are based on histone modification (*writing*).[142] A patented formulation that enhances expression of metallothionein proteins has been used to enhance antioxidant protection for bipolar patients. Other early epigenetic therapies include (a) methionine or SAMe supplements that inhibit serotonin reuptake by reducing expression of SERT transporter proteins, (b) folate/B12 supplements that reduce dopamine activity by enhanced expression of dopamine transporter proteins (DATs), and (c) histone modification therapies that regulate methylation and acetylation at histone tails. Future development of epigenetic bipolar disorder therapies appears highly promising, especially when specific *reading* and *erasing* therapies become available for this illness.

Bipolar Disorder – Triggered by DNA Damage?

Daily changes in the environment and diet produce minor epigenetic variations in gene expressions that are quite transient and may be imperceptible. Many transient epigenetic effects are caused by easily reversible histone modifications that may fade away in a few hours. However, gradually accumulating DNA damage, perhaps aggravated by severe physical or emotional trauma, may trigger onset of a permanent mental or physical illness. The relatively new science of epigenetics is making vast advances in understanding aging, DNA damage, and the development of physical and mental disorders. While Down syndrome, Angelman syndrome, Prader-Willi syndrome (PWS), and other germline genetic conditions are evident at birth, most forms of cancer and heart disease are epigenetic in nature and develop due to progressive DNA damage that changes the quality or production rate of expressed proteins. A recipe for cancer appears to be genetic predisposition followed by damage to key genes after birth. For example, breast cancer often involves germline mutations in *BRCA*, a family of DNA repair genes, followed by damage to additional pro-cancer genes with age.[143] An important question is whether DNA damage and resulting impairments in gene expression are primary factors in late-onset development of bipolar disorder.

There is increasing evidence that DNA damage is responsible for the onset of various illnesses such as schizophrenia, autism, post-traumatic stress disorder (PTSD), and other late-onset disorders; this is a subject of considerable debate.[144] The following discussion examines the possibility that bipolar onset has a strong epigenetic component involving loss of DNA integrity. Many researchers have suggested that bipolar disorder may be an epigenetic DNA-damage illness due to the frequent cases of sudden onset after years of excellent mental health.[145,146] Bipolar disorder's median age of onset is 25 years, indicating that germline genetic predisposition alone is not sufficient to produce the illness in most children and adolescents. Several plausible theories have attempted to explain the delayed onset feature of this mental illness. For decades, mainstream psychiatry blamed bipolar disorder's late onset on trauma associated with leaving the family unit.[147] Others have suggested that hormonal changes during puberty may have neurotransmission impacts that lead to bipolar disorder.[148] A respected recent theory has pointed to neuronal pruning that may have gone wrong after puberty.[149] For this study, I examined the possibility that bipolar disorder has a major epigenetic component involving adverse changes in gene expression caused by progressive DNA damage. Typical characteristics of a late-onset stable DNA-damage disorder include the following factors:

- Many cases of sudden onset after years of relative wellness
- Persistence after onset, indicating a life-changing event has occurred
- Violation of classic laws of Mendelian genetics
- A complex condition due to expression changes in numerous genes
- Elevated oxidative stress that accelerates assault on DNA
- Major emotional or physical trauma prior to onset

I evaluated each of these factors to assess if deviant epigenetic changes in gene expression are a likely trigger for bipolar disorder onset.

Sudden Onset: Most of the 1,500 bipolar families in my clinical database reported onset began in late adolescence or early adulthood with many cases having a sudden appearance of symptoms. I have met hundreds of bipolar patients who reported a history of high accomplishment prior to a massive change in mental functioning that developed in just a few days or weeks.

Persistence after Onset: Epigenetic disorders can persist indefinitely following deviant changes in gene expression that are not fixed by DNA repair. Bipolar disorder generally doesn't go away after onset despite the multitude of aggressive therapies over the years, meeting this criterion for a DNA-damage role. After onset, most bipolar patients are challenged by the illness for the rest of their life. Clinical therapies to reverse DNA damage are under development but are not yet available.

Mendelian Genetics: As described in Chapter 1, bipolar disorder runs very strongly in families with higher heritability than observed in depression, schizophrenia, and other major mental illnesses. Although this condition has a strong genetic component, the concordance in identical twins is less than 100%, which violates classic laws of Mendelian genetics. The genetic aspects of bipolar disorder are discussed in more detail in Chapter 8.

Bipolar Disorder Complexity: Cancer and other major DNA-damage disorders are inherently complex since a major loss of DNA integrity can permanently alter the expression of numerous genes, not just a single gene. The impact for each person depends on several factors that include their unique combination of inborn and acquired mutated genes. Clinicians and researchers differ on many aspects of bipolar disorder, but virtually all agree on the high degree of complexity of the condition.[150]

Oxidative Overload: Dozens of published bipolar disorder studies indicate excessive oxidative stress and inflammation are associated with the illness.[151] As mentioned in Chapters 1 and 2, my chemistry database for 1,500 bipolar patients indicated that 95% of them exhibited markers for very significant oxidative overload and inflammation. There is little doubt that elevated oxidative stress is a distinctive feature of bipolar disorder, thus it meets another criterion for an epigenetic DNA-damage disorder.

Trauma: Medical histories for our bipolar disorder population reveal a very high incidence of major trauma at the time of onset. In my experience, the most common adverse event is the collapse of a love relationship. Other patients developed the disorder soon after an auto accident, basic training, joining a religious seminary, physical injury, severe illness, academic failure, or other stressful events. Human and animal studies show that emotional trauma can permanently impair function of the amygdala, hippocampus, and prefrontal cortex, as well as altering cortisol and norepinephrine activity. For more than a century, psychiatry has known that severe trauma, especially in childhood, can contribute to a mental disorder.[152,153] We now have strong evidence that this may represent more than troubling memories with psychological impacts, but also permanent changes in gene expression, brain biochemistry, and neurotransmission.

Conclusion: Each of the above criteria for DNA-damage onset was met for bipolar disorder, and this was important to this investigation. Although not 100% proven, this indicates that bipolar disorder involves the combination of (a) strong genetic predisposition followed by (b) subsequent loss of DNA integrity that alters composition of expressed proteins or abnormal rates of delivery to cells. Our ability to protect genomic integrity depends on DNA repair capability and proper expression of protective antioxidant proteins. Genetic weakness in these protections likely contribute to the strong heritability of bipolar disorder. I conclude that the risk for bipolar disorder likely includes both inborn vulnerability for neurotransmission dysregulation, as well as weakness in protecting DNA integrity.

References

129. Wu, C. T., & Morris, J. R. (2001). Genes, genetics, and epigenetics: a correspondence. *Science, 293*(5532), 1103–1105.
130. Wu, T., Cai, W., & Chen, X. (2023). Epigenetic regulation of neurotransmitter signaling in neurological disorders. *Neurobiology of Disease, 184*, 106232.
131. Bannister, A. J., & Kouzarides, T. (2011). Regulation of chromatin by histone modifications. *Cell research, 21*(3), 381–395.
132. Guo, J. (2014). Transcription: the epicenter of gene expression. *Journal of Zhejiang University SCIENCE B, 15*, 409–411.
133. Catalanotto, C., Cogoni, C., & Zardo, G. (2016). MicroRNA in control of gene expression: an overview of nuclear functions. *International journal of molecular sciences, 17*(10), 1712.
134. Alles, J., Fehlmann, T., Fischer, U., Backes, C., Galata, V., Minet, M., ... & Meese, E. (2019). An estimate of the total number of true human miRNAs. *Nucleic acids research, 47*(7), 3353–3364.
135. Biswas, S., & Rao, C. M. (2018). Epigenetic tools (The Writers, The Readers and The Erasers) and their implications in cancer therapy. *European journal of pharmacology, 837*, 8–24.
136. Esteve-Puig, R., Bueno-Costa, A., & Esteller, M. (2020). Writers, readers and erasers of RNA modifications in cancer. *Cancer letters, 474*, 127–137.
137. Chi, P., Allis, C. D., & Wang, G. G. (2010). Covalent histone modifications—miswritten, misinterpreted and mis-erased in human cancers. *Nature reviews cancer, 10*(7), 457–469.

138. Mio, C., Bulotta, S., Russo, D., & Damante, G. (2019). Reading cancer: chromatin readers as druggable targets for cancer treatment. *Cancers, 11*(1), 61.

139. Pérez-Salvia, M., & Esteller, M. (2017). Bromodomain inhibitors and cancer therapy: From structures to applications. *Epigenetics, 12*(5), 323–339.

140. Ho, P. T., Clark, I. M., & Le, L. T. (2022). MicroRNA-based diagnosis and therapy. *International journal of molecular sciences, 23*(13), 7167.

141. He, B., Zhao, Z., Cai, Q., Zhang, Y., Zhang, P., Shi, S., ... & Wang, X. (2020). miRNA-based biomarkers, therapies, and resistance in Cancer. *International journal of biological sciences, 16*(14), 2628.

142. Ludwig, B., & Dwivedi, Y. (2016). Dissecting bipolar disorder complexity through epigenomic approach. *Molecular psychiatry, 21*(11), 1490–1498.

143. Welcsh, P. L., & King, M. C. (2001). BRCA1 and BRCA2 and the genetics of breast and ovarian cancer. *Human molecular genetics, 10*(7), 705–713.

144. Shiwaku, H., & Okazawa, H. (2015). Impaired DNA damage repair as a common feature of neurodegenerative diseases and psychiatric disorders. *Current molecular medicine, 15*(2), 119–128.

145. Ranjecar, P. K., Hinge, A., et al. (2003). Decreased antioxidant enzymes and membrane essential polyunsaturated fatty acids in schizophrenic and bipolar mood disorder patients. *Psychiatry Research, 121*, 109–122.

146. Andreazza, A. C., Frey, B. N., Erdtmann, B., Salvador, M., Rombaldi, F., Santin, A., ... & Kapczinski, F. (2007). DNA damage in bipolar disorder. *Psychiatry Research, 153*(1), 27–32.

147. Hatfield, A. B. (1992). Leaving home: Separation issues in psychiatric illness. *Psychosocial Rehabilitation Journal, 15*(4), 37.

148. Saugstad, L. F. (1989). Mental illness and cognition in relation to age at puberty: a hypothesis. *Clinical Genetics, 36*(3), 156–167.

149. Smart, K., & Boileau, I. (2023). Uncovering the link between synaptic density and mental illness through in vivo imaging. *Journal of Psychiatry and Neuroscience, 48*(2), E143-E148.

150. Ludwig, B., & Dwivedi, Y. (2016). Dissecting bipolar disorder complexity through epigenomic approach. *Molecular psychiatry, 21*(11), 1490–1498.

151. Yirün, M. C., Kübranur, Ü. N. A. L., Şen, N. A., Yirün, O., Aydemir, Ç., & Erol, G. Ö. K. A. (2016). Evaluation of oxidative stress in bipolar disorder in terms of total oxidant status, total antioxidant status, and oxidative stress index. *Archives of Neuropsychiatry, 53*(3), 194.

152. Park, Y. M., Shekhtman, T., & Kelsoe, J. R. (2020). Interaction between adverse childhood experiences and polygenic risk in patients with bipolar disorder. *Translational psychiatry, 10*(1), 326.

153. Aas, M., Henry, C., Andreassen, O. A., Bellivier, F., Melle, I., & Etain, B. (2016). The role of childhood trauma in bipolar disorders. *International journal of bipolar disorders, 4*, 1–10.

CHAPTER 8

Advances in Genetics Research

Collaborating Genes and Bipolar Disorder

As science advances, the detailed functional role of every gene will be revealed. Some genes work alone and perform a single task. For example, the SERT gene's primary job is to produce serotonin transporter proteins that enable reuptake. However, many genes collaborate with hundreds of others to enable complex processes, such as cardiovascular function, neurotransmission, or immunity. A great advantage of multigene processes is redundancy, since a single mutated or otherwise weakened gene may not cause great harm. In addition, a multitude of collaborating genes may confer necessary complexity of function. Unfortunately, high complexity disorders can also present great difficulties when serious problems develop. It is difficult to diagnose and treat a complex disorder if there are many combinations of genetic and epigenetic mutations that may be responsible. This has been especially challenging in bipolar disorder because the brain changes that cause alternating mania and depression have remained unknown.

Late-Onset Mental Disorders: While Down syndrome and other developmental disorders are evident soon after birth, severe mental disorders typically develop after puberty. Major depressive disorder, schizophrenia, and bipolar disorder often appear quite suddenly after many years of relative normality. Most delayed onset illnesses involve inborn gene mutations that do not disrupt health until continuing DNA damage contributes additional gene malfunctions. The timing and severity of this damage depends not only on toxic environments or physical/mental trauma but also on the individual's DNA repair and antioxidant capabilities, which are largely genetic. This complicates the search for the essence of bipolar disorder because predisposing genes likely include numerous DNA-damage factors that may have little or no direct relevance to mania/depression cycling and the bipolar disorder syndrome.

As described in Chapters 1 and 2, bipolar disorder exhibits unusually strong heritability compared to other mental disorders. In a major surprise, researchers were unable to find any gene directly associated with the condition during the first 30 years of careful genetic studies. This revealed bipolar disorder as a highly complex condition involving a great number of low-effect predisposing gene variants. Many hundreds of genes collaborate to enable relatively stable neuronal behavior during normal mental functioning. It appears bipolar disorder may involve inborn genetic weakness in this gene "team" that becomes more severe due to additional gene impairments that develop with age. The result could be loss of neuronal stability and a tendency for chronic switching between mania and depression. In recent years, researchers have sought to identify the elusive bipolar gene variants in the hope they might shed light on this mysterious mental illness.

Genome-Wide Association Studies

A recent breakthrough has been the Human Genome Project (HGP) and improvements in genotyping technology that have led to large genome-wide association studies (GWAS) capable of identifying low-effect susceptibility genes. Large population GWAS experiments are underway for bipolar disorder, schizophrenia, cancer, and several other heritable disorders. This effort typically involves scanning the entire genome for genetic variants producing the ability to simultaneously identify many thousands of SNP mutations. Since the year 2000, GWAS researchers have compared the DNA of bipolar patients and nonbipolar controls in a search for predisposing gene variants. Two early bipolar disorder studies involved fewer than 2,500 cases and failed to yield significant results.[154,155] However, a larger mega-analysis study of 4,387 cases and 6,209 controls found the first genome-wide significant association: the *ANK3* (ankyrin G) gene, with a highly significant p-value of 9.1 x 10^{-9}.[156] This finding was replicated by three subsequent studies. Another early bipolar susceptibility gene was the *CACNA1C* variant that has become the subject of many research studies.[157] Since that time, improved genetics technology and larger population studies have gradually identified additional bipolar gene variants, and this number reached 31 in year 2017[158] and increased to a total of 64 in 2021.[159] These GWAS findings became a major component of this investigation.

Exclusion Analysis of GWAS Gene Variants

GWAS identification of predisposing bipolar disorder genes presents a promising opportunity to achieve better understanding of the causes and mechanisms of this unique mental illness. Although more than a thousand gene mutations may predispose to bipolar disorder, scientists are eagerly studying early known variants in a search for clues to the etiology and treatment opportunities for this elusive mental illness. It was exciting to learn in 2017 that GWAS had identified 32 pro-bipolar gene variants, including two in the *ERBB2* gene. Like thousands of others, I studied what was known about these genes with respect to functional roles and potential impairments resulting from these mutations. However, the presence of DNA-damage genes complicates the search for gene variants that relate directly to bipolar disorder and mania/depression switching. There are at least three major components to the heritability of bipolar disorder, and each involves large collaborating gene teams that may be weakened at birth.

- Gene variants that directly relate to the bipolar disorder syndrome
- Impaired antioxidant protection genes
- Impaired DNA repair genes

To address this problem, I developed an exclusion analysis approach that disregards DNA repair and oxidative protection genes that may be obscuring the search for true bipolar disorder genes. Excluded genes in this analysis included those strongly associated with cancer, fatty acid damage, and other conditions dominated by DNA damage. For example, the *ERBB2* gene with two pro-bipolar variants is strongly implicated in lung, breast, and leukemia cancers.[160] I also evaluated dozens of known blood-brain barrier genes since their variants could contribute to DNA damage, but none were found in the 31 GWAS bipolar-risk genes.

I was surprised to learn that the majority of the 32 gene variants were associated with increased cancer risk, including several that are major cancer genes. These genes and others strongly associated with DNA damage were removed from this analysis to identify variants more likely to be directly associated with bipolar disorder. This approach is somewhat arbitrary due to incomplete knowledge of the functional roles of many of these genes. Some excluded genes may also relate directly to bipolar disorder, or certain accepted genes may have unknown roles in DNA damage. The criteria used in making exclusion decisions is described in Appendix C. The predisposing genes identified in 2017 represent a small percentage of the bipolar variant population. On the other hand, the GWAS gene variants represent relatively strong bipolar disorder risk factors due to the higher frequency of appearance that enabled their discovery. Overall, this approach appeared to offer the best available opportunity to identify true bipolar disorder genes based on the 2017 GWAS findings.

The exclusion analysis results are summarized as follows: A total of 22 bipolar variants were excluded due to close association with genomic damage. The 10 remaining genes (shown in Figure 14) are assumed to entail higher probability of direct relevance to the essence of bipolar disorder. The functions of the 10 "bipolar genes" were carefully examined for any roles in neurotransmission or regulation of neuronal activity. Major functions of the 10 misbehaving bipolar genes are summarized below:

> *ANK3*: This was the first bipolar gene variant identified in high-population genetics studies and is regarded as a relatively strong contributor to bipolar disorder risk compared to other small-effect variants. *ANK3* encodes an adaptor protein (ankyrin-G) that regulates the positioning of voltage-gated ion channels including placement of high concentrations of voltage-gated Na^+ channels at AIS and nodes of Ranvier.[161]

> *CACNA1C*: This gene expresses L-type voltage-gated calcium channels that open during depolarization causing an inrush of Ca^{++} ions that trigger the ejection of neurotransmitters into a synapse. It also has a key role in activating K^+ channels during repolarization (recovery from an action potential), along with numerous other important roles in neurotransmission.[162]

ADCY2: This gene encodes for members of the adenylate cyclase family that catalyze formation of second messenger cAMP at dendrite receptors, thus having a major impact on several neurotransmission systems.[163] *ADCY2* also mediates Ca^{++} processes in neurons and glial cells.

SCN2A: This gene encodes for $Na_v1.2$ voltage-gated Na^+ ion channels. Missense and loss-of-function mutations in $Na_v1.2$ impair the excitability of GABAergic inhibitory neurons and are associated with neuronal hyperexcitability and several forms of epilepsy.[164]

GRIN2A: This gene codes for an NMDA receptor subunit, and its variants are implicated in 85% of all forms of epilepsy. The molecular functions include glutamate-gated calcium channel activity, beta amyloid binding, and zinc ion binding.[165]

ZnF592: Encodes a zinc-finger transcription factor that regulates expression in the cerebellum and substantia nigra (site of dopamine neurons), along with other roles in the periphery (outside the brain). It is also associated with two forms of superoxide dismutase (SOD) that protect DNA and was accepted for this analysis with reservations.[166]

WFDC12: Encodes a protease inhibitor that tends to increase the half-life of expressed proteins. While an SNP-weakened *WFDC12* variant could increase DNA damage, it appears to have a greater effect on ion channel behavior and regulation of neuronal activity.[167]

LMAN2L: Encodes VIP36 proteins that are components of vesicle and neuron membranes. They have a role in the formation of receptors and may interact with *ANK3* in placement of ion channels.[168]

MRPS33: Encodes a component of mitochondrial ribosome proteins that have a major role in translation and protein synthesis. At least one variant can cause epilepsy (neuronal hyperactivity). Despite evidence of increased lung cancer risk, *MRPS33* was accepted for this analysis with reservations.[169]

PACS1: *PACS1* plays a role in localizing neuron, vesicle, and glia membrane proteins, and this gene assists in ion channel regulation. Mutated PACS1 proteins are associated with several neurodevelopmental disorders. *PACS1* overexpression is associated with reduced density of dendritic spines.[170]

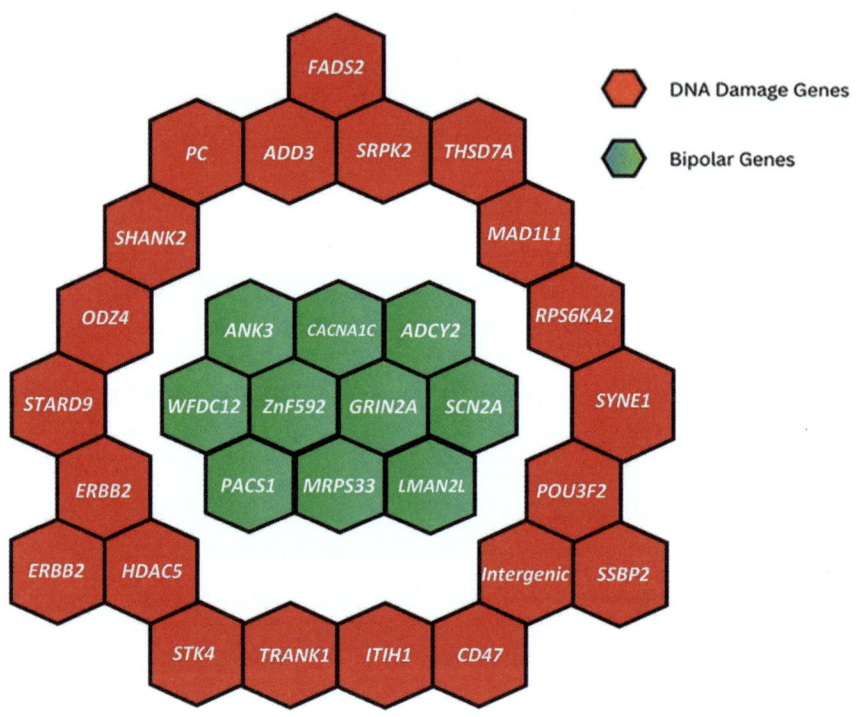

Figure 14. Exclusion Analysis Results (GWAS 2017)

The majority of the "accepted" genes are associated with formation, placement, or behavior of ion channels, including the intensively studied *ANK3* and *CACNA1A* variants. *ANK3* has a major role in the placement of Na+ voltage-gated ion channels that open to initiate neuron firing. Misbehaving Ca++ channels have a direct influence on K+ outflow during action potentials, and bipolar disorder has been associated with elevated Ca++ cytosol concentrations in neurons. Other accepted genes were found to have roles in localization (positioning) of ion channels or neuronal hyperactivity. This early evidence strongly suggests that misbehaving ion channels are central to the genetic risk for bipolar disorder. This result is not surprising since ion channels are responsible for resting voltages, neuronal excitability, and the kinetics of neurotransmission. For several years, many researchers have suggested that impaired ion channel functioning may represent a dominant factor in bipolar disorder. For example, a 2014 review article by Judy and Zandl presented strong evidence that bipolar disorder may be a channelopathy.[171] Although not 100% proven, I concluded that ion channel gene mutations represent the primary genetic predisposition for bipolar disorder, and in May 2018, I presented this theory at the American Psychiatric Association Annual Meeting in New York City.

Additional GWAS Variants (2021): Continuing genome-wide studies are providing remarkable new insights into the underlying neurobiology of several major mental disorders. In June 2021, a *Nature Genetics* article[159] identified an additional 32 bipolar disorder variants, bringing the total to 64. I evaluated the new information using the exclusion analysis approach, and the results are displayed in Figure 15. In summary, 27 of the 32 variants were closely associated with DNA damage, with just 5 new variants suspected of direct relevance to the bipolar disorder syndrome:

> *CACNB2*: This gene encodes a subunit of voltage-gated calcium channels that are primary factors in action potentials and neurotransmission.[172]

> *KCNB1*: This gene encodes for the $K_v2.1$ ion channel that is the major contributor to delayed rectifier K^+ currents needed for rapid repolarization.[173]

> *HOMER1*: This versatile gene regulates glutamate synapses and enables activation of calcium ion channels.[174,175]

> *MDFIC2*: Encodes proteins that act as a transcriptional activator or repressor for viral genome expression with impacts on immune function. At this writing, this gene variant's role in increasing bipolar disorder risk is unknown.[176]

> *RP1-84015.2 lincRNA*: This gene encodes RNA proteins, and this variant has been implicated in muscular dystrophy, bipolar disorder,

schizophrenia, and ADHD. At this writing, the variant's specific role in mental illness risk is unclear.[159]

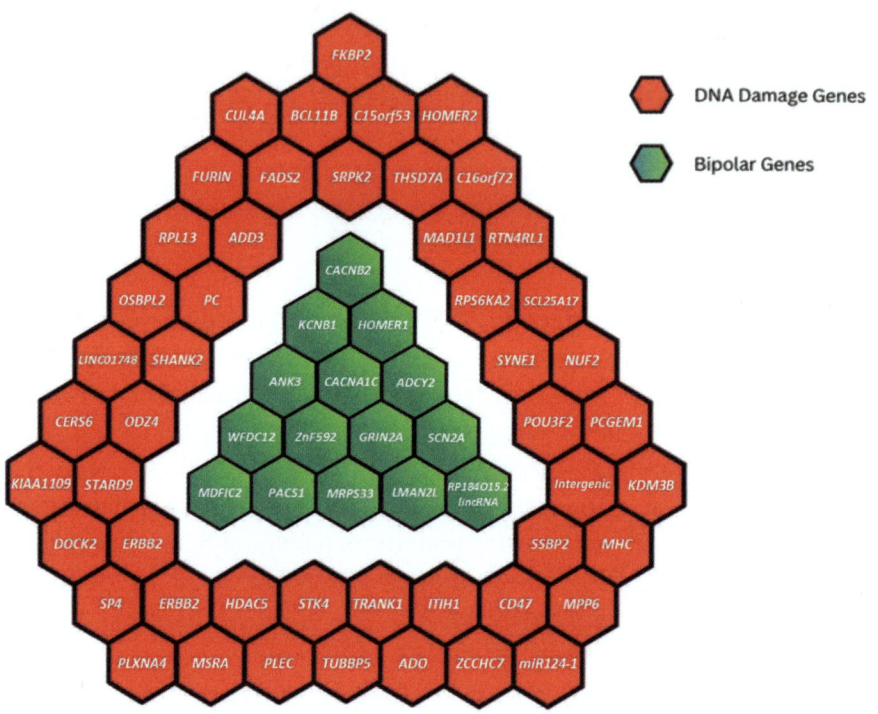

Figure 15. Exclusion Analysis Results (2021)

Bipolar Disorder Genetic Predispositions

The exclusion analysis of the 64 bipolar disorder variants has identified 15 mutated genes that appear directly related to bipolar disorder while the others have prominent roles in DNA damage. More than 60% of the bipolar variants involve K$^+$ and Ca^{++} channels that are key factors in neurotransmission, and several others have roles in regulation of neuronal activity. The 2021 GWAS findings are consistent with those reported in 2017. The high percentage of ion channel variants after excluding DNA-damage genes is strong evidence that mutated ion-channel genes represent the primary genetic risk (and perhaps the cause) for bipolar disorder. However, the discovery that about 75% of GWAS pro-bipolar variants involve cancer and other DNA-damage genes was a surprise that cannot be dismissed. Their prominent presence suggests that a pronounced genetic weakness in protecting DNA integrity may be an essential factor in the development of bipolar disorder.

Evidence of Extreme DNA Damage in Bipolar Disorder: As previously mentioned, loss of DNA integrity is the reason we age, and we are learning that unrepaired DNA damage may be a primary cause of cancer, heart disease, mental disorders, and numerous other late-onset maladies.[177] The discovery that DNA-damage genes dominate known bipolar variants suggests that a genetic tendency for severe DNA damage may be a prerequisite for bipolar disorder. If this is true, bipolar populations should exhibit evidence of accelerated aging and greater incidence of diseases that are unrelated to bipolar disorder. A review of the scientific literature reveals this is exactly the case. For example, the risk of dying from heart disease in bipolar patients may be twice that of the general population.[178] Some studies indicate the risk for multiple sclerosis is two times higher, diabetes three times higher, and breast cancer 30% higher.[179,180,181] Patients with bipolar disorder exhibit an increased frequency of gastrointestinal tract illnesses, immune disorders, migraines, liver disease, kidney failure, and many other illnesses. Life expectancy of patients diagnosed with bipolar disorder is disturbingly low throughout the world, far beyond that attributed to suicide risk. The median age at death is 67 years compared to 79 years in the general population.[182] It seems terribly unfair that most bipolar patients must endure poor general health and early death in addition to the daunting challenges of mania and depression. This may help explain bipolar disorder's remarkably high suicide rate described in Chapter 1. In summary, there is very strong evidence of unusually severe DNA damage in bipolar disorder.

The Apparent Cause of Bipolar Disorder: Bipolar disorder's inborn weaknesses (mutations) in the ion channel team are not sufficient to cause significant symptoms in early childhood. However, additional DNA damage over many years likely triggers onset of the illness. There are more than 250 known DNA repair genes that collaborate to minimize the constant and relentless injuries to our precious DNA molecules.[183] This DNA-repair gene team typically has thousands of SNP variants with various impacts, and many people are born with relative weakness in this protective system. In addition, there are more than 60 major antioxidant protection genes and hundreds of associated transcription factors that combat free radical assault on DNA, and many people are born with weakness in these mechanisms as well.[184] All humans depend on these protective genes that guard against early onset of health problems. However, recent cancer research indicates that major ion channel impairments weaken DNA damage repair (DDR) and are associated with accelerated DNA damage.[185,186] This suggests bipolar disorder and other channelopathies are intrinsically prone to severe rates of DNA damage due to this additional assault on DNA integrity.

I conclude that the principal cause of bipolar disorder is genetic predisposition for two coincident factors:

- Genetic Weakness in the Team of Collaborating Ion Channel Genes.

- Genetic Tendency for Accelerated DNA Damage.

References

154. The Wellcome Trust Case Control Consortium. (2007). Genome-wide association study of 14,000 cases of seven common diseases and 3,000 shared controls. *Nature, 447*(7145), 661–678.

155. Sklar, P., Smoller, J. W., Fan, J., Ferreira, M. A. R., Perlis, R. H., Chambert, K., ... & Purcell, S. M. (2008). Whole-genome association study of bipolar disorder. *Molecular psychiatry, 13*(6), 558–569.

156. Ferreira M. A., O'Donovan M. C., et al. (2008) Collaborative genome-wide association analysis supports a role for ANK3 and CACNA1C in bipolar disorder. *Nature Genetics 40*, 1056–1058.

157. Bigos, K. L., Mattay, V. S., Callicott, J. H., Straub, R. E., Vakkalanka, R., Kolachana, B., ... & Weinberger, D. R. (2010). Genetic variation in CACNA1C affects brain circuitries related to mental illness. *Archives of general psychiatry, 67*(9), 939–945.

158. Stahl, E. A., Breen, G., Forstner, A. J., McQuillin, A., Ripke, S., Trubetskoy, V., ... & Reif, A. (2019). Genome-wide association study identifies 30 loci associated with bipolar disorder. *Nature genetics, 51*(5), 793–803.

159. Mullins, N., Forstner, A. J., O'Connell, K. S., Coombes, B., Coleman, J. R., Qiao, Z., ... & Potash, J. B. (2021). Genome-wide association study of more than 40,000 bipolar disorder cases provides new insights into the underlying biology. *Nature genetics*, *53*(6), 817–829.

160. Kauraniemi, P., & Kallioniemi, A. (2006). Activation of multiple cancer-associated genes at the ERBB2 amplicon in breast cancer. *Endocrine-related cancer*, *13*(1), 39–49.

161. Yoon, S., Piguel, N. H., & Penzes, P. (2022). Roles and mechanisms of ankyrin-G in neuropsychiatric disorders. *Experimental & Molecular Medicine*, *54*(7), 867–877.

162. Moon, A. L., Haan, N., Wilkinson, L. S., Thomas, K. L., & Hall, J. (2018). CACNA1C: association with psychiatric disorders, behavior, and neurogenesis. *Schizophrenia bulletin*, *44*(5), 958–965.

163. National Library of Medicine (2004). *ADCY2: adenylate cyclase 2 (Homo Sapiens (human).* https://www.ncbi.nlm.nih.gov/gene?Db=gene&Cmd=DetailsSearch&Term=108

164. Wolff, M., Brunklaus, A., & Zuberi, S. M. (2019). Phenotypic spectrum and genetics of SCN 2A-related disorders, treatment options, and outcomes in epilepsy and beyond. *Epilepsia*, *60*, S59-S67.

165. Shepard, N., Baez-Nieto, D., Iqbal, S., Kurganov, E., Budnik, N., Campbell, A. J., ... & Farsi, Z. (2024). Differential functional consequences of GRIN2A mutations associated with schizophrenia and neurodevelopmental disorders. *Scientific reports*, *14*(1), 2798.

166. Nicolas, E., Poitelon, Y., Chouery, E., Salem, N., Levy, N., Mégarbané, A., & Delague, V. (2010). CAMOS, a nonprogressive, autosomal recessive, congenital cerebellar ataxia, is caused by a mutant zinc-finger protein, ZNF592. *European journal of human genetics*, *18*(10), 1107–1113.

167. Li, G., Gu, L., Zhao, F., Hu, Y., Wang, X., Zeng, F., ... & Li, J. (2023). WFDC12-overexpressing contributes to the development of atopic dermatitis via accelerating ALOX12/15 metabolism and PAF accumulation. *Cell Death & Disease*, *14*(3), 185.

168. Alkhater, R. A., Wang, P., Ruggieri, A., Israelian, L., Walker, S., Scherer, S. W., ... & Minassian, B. A. (2019). Dominant LMAN2L mutation causes intellectual disability with remitting epilepsy. *Annals of Clinical and Translational Neurology*, *6*(4), 807–811.

169. Saada, A., Shaag, A., Arnon, S., Dolfin, T., Miller, C., Fuchs-Telem, D., ... & Elpeleg, O. (2007). Antenatal mitochondrial disease caused

by mitochondrial ribosomal protein (MRPS22) mutation. *Journal of medical genetics, 44*(12), 784–786.

170. Köttgen, M., Benzing, T., Simmen, T., Tauber, R., Buchholz, B., Feliciangeli, S., ... & Walz, G. (2005). Trafficking of TRPP2 by PACS proteins represents a novel mechanism of ion channel regulation. *The EMBO journal, 24*(4), 705–716.

171. Judy, J. T., & Zandi, P. P. (2013). A review of potassium channels in bipolar disorder. *Frontiers in genetics, 4,* 105.

172. Liu, F., Gong, X., Yao, X., Cui, L., Yin, Z., Li, C., ... & Wang, F. (2019). Variation in the CACNB2 gene is associated with functional connectivity of the Hippocampus in bipolar disorder. *BMC psychiatry, 19,* 1–7.

173. De Kovel, C. G., Syrbe, S., Brilstra, E. H., Verbeek, N., Kerr, B., Dubbs, H., ... & Koeleman, B. P. (2017). Neurodevelopmental disorders caused by de novo variants in KCNB1 genotypes and phenotypes. *JAMA neurology, 74*(10), 1228–1236.

174. Yoon, S., Piguel, N. H., Khalatyan, N., Dionisio, L. E., Savas, J. N., & Penzes, P. (2021). Homer1 promotes dendritic spine growth through ankyrin-G and its loss reshapes the synaptic proteome. *Molecular psychiatry, 26*(6), 1775–1789.

175. Worley, P. F., Zeng, W., Huang, G., Kim, J. Y., Shin, D. M., Kim, M. S., ... & Muallem, S. (2007). Homer proteins in Ca2+ signaling by excitable and non-excitable cells. *Cell calcium, 42*(4–5), 363–371.

176. National Library of Medicine. (2024). *MDFIC MyoD family inhibitor domain containing [Homo sapiens (human)].* https://www.ncbi.nlm. nih.gov/gene?Db=gene&Cmd=DetailsSearch&Term=29969

177. Lam, F. C. (2022). The DNA damage response-from cell biology to human disease. *J Transl Genet Genom, 6*(2), 204–222.

178. Swartz, H. A., & Fagiolini, A. (2012). Cardiovascular disease and bipolar disorder: risk and clinical implications. *J Clin Psychiatry, 73*(12), 1563–5.

179. Crump, C., Sundquist, K., Winkleby, M. A., & Sundquist, J. (2013). Comorbidities and mortality in bipolar disorder: a Swedish national cohort study. *JAMA psychiatry, 70*(9).

180. Young, A. H., & Grunze, H. (2013). Physical health of patients with bipolar disorder. *Acta Psychiatrica Scandinavica, 127,* 3–10.

181. Halstead, S., Cao, C., Mohr, G. H., Ebdrup, B. H., Pillinger, T., McCutcheon, R. A., ... & Warren, N. (2024). Prevalence of multimorbidity in people with and without severe mental illness: a

systematic review and meta-analysis. *The Lancet Psychiatry*, *11*(6), 431–442.

182. Chan, J. K. N., Tong, C. H. Y., Wong, C. S. M., Chen, E. Y. H., & Chang, W. C. (2022). Life expectancy and years of potential life lost in bipolar disorder: systematic review and meta-analysis. *The British Journal of Psychiatry*, *221*(3), 567–576.

183. Olivieri, M., Cho, T., Álvarez-Quilón, A., Li, K., Schellenberg, M. J., Zimmermann, M., ... & Durocher, D. (2020). A genetic map of the response to DNA damage in human cells. *Cell*, *182*(2), 481–496.

184. Gelain, D. P., Dalmolin, R. J., Belau, V. L., Moreira, J. C., Klamt, F., & Castro, M. A. (2009). A systematic review of human antioxidant genes. *Frontiers in Bioscience*, *14*(12), 4457–4463.

185. Girault, A., & Brochiero, E. (2014). Evidence of K+ channel function in epithelial cell migration, proliferation, and repair. *American Journal of Physiology-Cell Physiology*, *306*(4), C307-C319.

186. Maliszewska-Olejniczak, K., & Bednarczyk, P. (2024). Novel insights into the role of ion channels in cellular DNA damage response. *Mutation Research-Reviews in Mutation Research*, *793*, 108488.

CHAPTER 9

A Search for the Switching Mechanism

Introduction

While it was important to identify ion channel impairments and DNA damage as central to bipolar disorder, an explanation for the unique mania/depression switching phenomenon was still missing in this investigation. Beginning in late 2017, I began a search for ion channel impairments that could compromise stability of neuronal activity and cause mania/depression cycling. The unique chronic cycling between mania and depression distinguishes bipolar disorder from all other psychiatric disorders. This core aspect of the illness has been researched for more than a century with very little progress in understanding its cause or mechanisms. For example, a 1998 theory[187] suggested that bipolar cycling results from alternate domination by brain hemispheres in which one fosters mania and the other depression. Like most switching theories prior to the year 2000, this theory encountered a disappointing lack of supporting evidence. A major barrier to switching research has been powerful medications consumed by the vast majority of bipolar patients that can blur the results.[188] Many treatment-emergent affective switch (TEAS) studies have examined the mechanisms of medications that can induce or eliminate mania or depression, but none have convincingly explained the tendency for chronic cycling between mania and depression.[189] The century-old search for the cause of mania/depression switching has been called the "holy grail" of bipolar disorder. A comprehensive 2010 review article[190] stated that the causes and mechanisms of bipolar disorder switching were still unknown. Magioncalda and Martino recently published a model that includes a plausible but somewhat incomplete explanation for both cause and mechanisms.[191] They hypothesized that immune-mediated white matter impairments cause limbic-network damage that destabilizes neurotransmission. They suggested this may cause unidentified perturbations that impair regulation of serotonin or dopamine systems and trigger chronic mania/ depression transitions. Australians Berk and colleagues have published a hypothesis that bipolar disorder switching results from dopamine dysregulation and presented considerable evidence to support this model.[192,193] These two studies are among the most detailed and persuasive published theories of bipolar disorder switching at this writing. However, this investigation's discovery that misbehaving ion channels and heightened DNA damage are central to bipolar disorder presented a great advantage in the search for the cause of mania/ depression cycling. My search for the elusive switching mechanism concentrated exclusively on ion channel impairments and accelerated DNA damage, based on the following model:

- Hundreds of ion channel genes collaborate to enable stability of neuronal firing in healthy brains.

- Inborn weaknesses in this ion channel team predispose to bipolar disorder, but they usually are not sufficient to produce onset of the illness during childhood or adolescence.

- Increasing DNA damage with advancing age eventually contributes new ion channel or other impairments that disrupt neuronal stability and lead to mania/depression switching. In the absence of successful treatment, this switching tendency may be permanent.

There are many thousands of gene mutation combinations that could weaken the family of collaborating ion channel genes and predispose to bipolar disorder. Each ion channel gene has dozens of potential SNPs that may or may not significantly impact function. To complicate matters, an individual variant may cause either loss of function or gain of function. The multitude of variant combinations that might trigger onset explains (a) the absence of a dominant bipolar risk gene and (b) the disorder's heterogeneity (great variation of symptoms and traits for individual patients). It is quite remarkable that most of us are born with healthy brains that function adequately despite thousands of things that can and do go wrong. An important feature of good mental health is the collective ability of our 80 billion brain neurons to minimize spurious hyperactivity or hypoactivity as we live each day. Epilepsy and panic attacks are neuronal hyperactivity disorders in which misbehaving neurotransmitters have been identified, and generally effective treatments are available. In contrast, classic bipolar disorder involves chronic transitions between neuronal hyperactivity (mania) and a unique form of depression, and the cause and brain mechanisms have remained unknown. Although today's treatments typically provide partial improvement, most patients with bipolar disorder continue to experience an unacceptable quality of life. Identifying the cause and mechanisms of mania/depression switching may be essential to development of improved treatment outcomes and prevention strategies.

An Early Focus on Neuronal Hyperactivity and Mania

The majority of our 1,500+ patient bipolar population reported their primary symptom at onset was mania or hypomania that gradually increased in severity, typically followed by a switch to depression. In my clinical experience, whenever a patient's mania came under good control, the tendency for serious depression seemed to disappear. Moreover, clinical improvements in the treatment of bipolar's depression phase rarely prevented the return of mania. These observations suggest that bipolar's depression episodes may be caused by mania. I decided to investigate whether progressive damage to ion channel genes might lead to a form of neuronal hyperactivity that could severely impair a neurotransmission system associated with clinical depression. My initial focus was on major neurotransmitter systems known to exhibit abnormal behavior in bipolar patients and have also been implicated in clinical depression. While serotonin, dopamine, norepinephrine, glutamate, and other transmitters may develop stable changes in activity after bipolar onset, one of them may develop out-of-control accelerating hyperactivity that eventually disables the system. This could neatly explain the abrupt switch to depression. This investigation's search for ion channel impairments that might produce nonstop increasing neuronal hyperactivity identified two leading possibilities: (a) potassium ion buildup outside neuronal membranes and (b) lost ability to form full resting voltages. This effort concentrated on these leading suspects in the hope they might explain the appearance of mania during bipolar disorder onset and lead to the switching mechanism.

Potassium Buildup Outside Neuron Membranes

Every neuron firing event involves rapid inward flow of Na^+ and Ca^{++} ions and outward flow of K^+ ions.[62,194] However, healthy neurons have the remarkable ability to quickly restore the original ion gradients and resting potentials because the actual amount of material transported is extremely small. When a neuron fires, voltage-gated Na^+, Ca^{++}, and K^+ channels open for only about a millisecond, and interior and exterior concentrations are nearly unaffected. Some neuroscientists refer to this tiny concentration change as "a drop in the ocean," which helps explain why some neurons can fire 200 times per second. Neuronal stability depends on the ability to restore ion gradients and resting voltage with extraordinary speed after an action potential. This ability is enabled by hundreds of special proteins expressed by ion channel genes. However, severe DNA damage to this collaborating gene team could prevent efficient clearance of potassium ions after neuron firing events. Scientists have known for years that elevated extracellular K^+ levels $(K^+)_o$ are associated with neuronal hyperactivity.[195] I decided to examine the possibility that mania/depression switching is triggered by lost ability to prevent potassium ion flooding outside certain severely impaired neurons. Potassium ion buildup outside neuronal membranes could be caused either by increased K^+ outflow or impaired clearance mechanisms. For example, excessive Ca^{++} cytosol concentrations would result in excessive K^+ flow rates through calcium-gated K^+ channels that might overwhelm clearance.

External potassium ion concentrations outside neurons are generally maintained at less than 3 mM/L (millimoles per liter) with the assistance of ion pumps at both neuronal and astrocyte membranes.[196] In addition, astrocyte glial cells assist potassium clearance by a mechanism called spatial buffering in which excess K^+ ions are removed like a vacuum cleaner inhaling dust particles.[197,198] Spatial buffering is mediated by inwardly rectifying Kir2 channels capable of rapid potassium clearance for $(K^+)_o$ concentrations exceeding 3 mM/L, but this capability ceases if levels surpass 15 mM/L. If $(K^+)_o$ levels escalate, excess potassium ions flow rapidly into astrocytes. Once inside the astrocyte network, tiny rivers of K^+ ions flow through glial gap junctions and are dumped into the bloodstream by astrocyte end-feet that wrap around brain capillaries. High K^+ conductance at the astrocyte end-feet enhances efficiency of spatial buffering. Some neurons are surrounded by astrocyte glial cells, while others exhibit a relatively sparse astrocyte population and are more vulnerable to potassium ion accumulations.

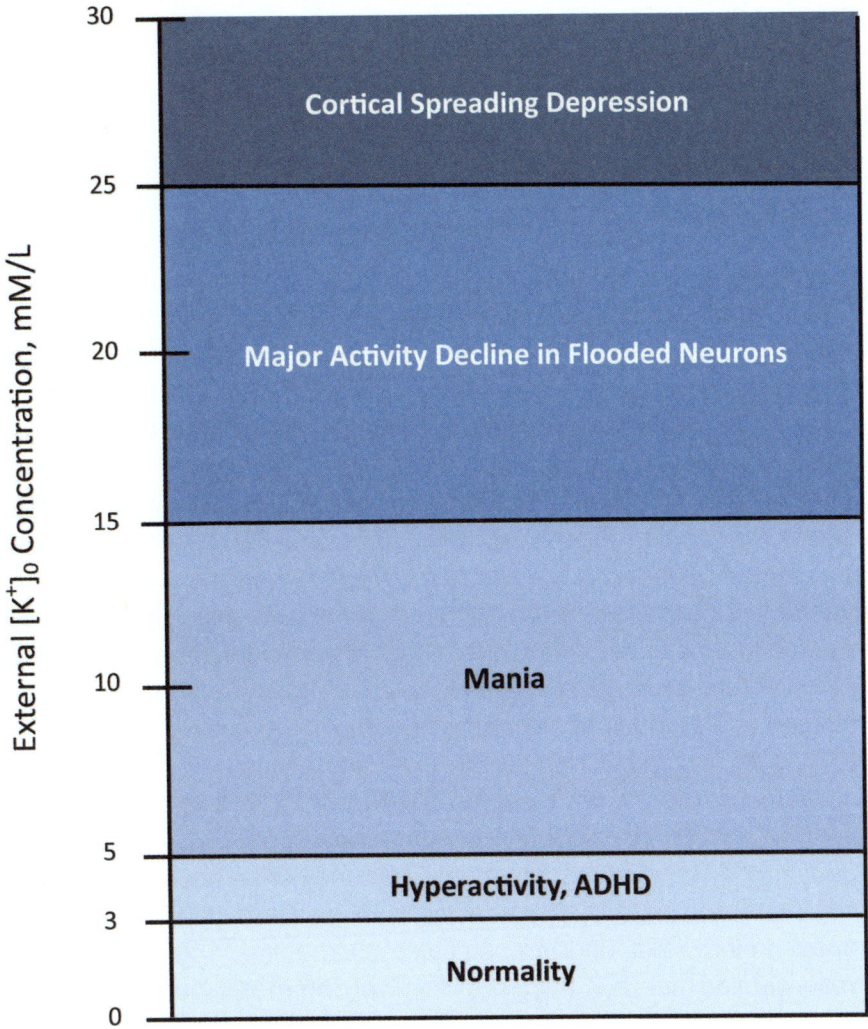

Figure 16. Effects of Elevated $(K^+)_o$ Levels

I soon learned that $(K^+)_o$ concentrations as high as 80 mM/L have been observed in research studies.[199,200] Scientific studies of cortical spreading depression (CSD) indicate that some brain sites shut down and nearly cease electrical activity when $(K^+)_o$ levels exceed 15 mM/L. Spreading depression refers to severely depressed neuronal activity that can quickly (and briefly) spread across neural tissues and likely is not related to bipolar depression. CSD provides an example of neuronal regions that are disabled during extreme elevations of extracellular potassium ions. Figure 16 shows some of the clinical effects associated with various $(K^+)_o$ elevations. Values between 3 and 5 mM/L are associated with ADHD and other hyperactivity conditions; mania typically involves levels above 5 mM/L, and epilepsy often exceeds 10 mM/L.[201] It is significant that $(K^+)_o$ levels above 15 mM/L could severely disable a neurotransmitter system and cause clinical depression.

Lost Ability to Develop Full Resting Neuron Voltages: A multitude of gene variant combinations could reduce resting potentials, including several not caused by impaired $(K^+)_o$ clearance mechanisms described in the previous section; for example, misplaced ion channel sites, dysregulated M currents, altered regulation by autoreceptors, and many other impairments. In another example, severe damage to ion channel genes after birth may alter K^+, Na^+, Ca^{++}, and Cl^- gradients and permeabilities that could reduce resting voltages (see Nernst and Goldman equations, Appendix A). Smaller rest voltages would increase neuronal hyperactivity because fewer excitatory neurotransmissions would be required to reach the threshold for firing. In summary, there are numerous ion channel impairments that could progressively shrink resting voltages and produce accelerating neuronal hyperactivity.

Expected Impacts on Neurotransmitters: The two mechanisms described above are closely related because both involve potassium flooding and reduced rest potentials, and they differ only in the underlying cause of neuronal hyperactivity. Regardless of causation, the impact on individual neurotransmitters is expected to be quite similar. While bipolar mania is known to involve dopamine, norepinephrine, glutamate, and other neurotransmitters, the transition to depression may involve a small fraction of brain sites (or a single site) experiencing especially severe impairments and loss of function. For this analysis, I arbitrarily assumed $(K^+)_o$ flooding would disable a single neurotransmitter system. A major challenge is that a proper bipolar disorder switching model requires the disabled transmitter system to recover and enable a transition back to mania, and this disqualified several potential switching mechanisms.

Discovery of a Promising Switching Mechanism

This book does not describe numerous failed attempts to identify the elusive switching mechanism. Success was finally achieved while evaluating the possibility that the switch to depression is triggered by extreme potassium ion flooding that severely disables a neurotransmitter system associated with clinical depression. This analysis was based on the following model:

1. Prior to bipolar onset, functional neuronal stability is achieved in the brain's major neurotransmitter systems despite significant genetic weakness in the team of 400+ ion channels.
2. Mania onset is caused by progressive (additional) DNA damage and ion channel impairments resulting in neuronal hyperactivity in several neurotransmitter systems.
3. While most transmitters may develop a stable degree of hyperactivity, it is assumed that one of them is damaged to the extent that it develops out-of-control buildup of extracellular potassium ions.
4. A mass-transfer analysis was employed to determine if severe potassium flooding and reduced resting potentials could seriously disable serotonin, dopamine, norepinephrine, or other transmitter systems, and trigger bipolar disorder's depression phase.

Transition to the Depression Phase: Potassium ion flooding would move resting voltage closer to threshold voltage, resulting in higher neuronal activity. This increased neuronal activity would cause an incrementally higher rate of K^+ ion outflow, with the new rate dependent on the specific combination of damaged ion channels. A neurotransmitter with excellent $(K^+)_o$ clearance might develop a stable degree of hyperactivity, while another might experience continuously increasing $(K^+)_o$ accumulations outside neuronal membranes. A mass-transport analysis indicated this could initiate a vicious cycle of accelerating K^+ ion outflow, reduced K^+ ion gradients, and shrinking resting voltages in a feedback loop. The $(K^+)_o$ increases may be very slow initially due to tiny incremental increases in K^+ outflow and slight reductions in resting voltage. This may help explain why mania and hypomania typically persist for several weeks or months before a transition to depression. In the absence of effective treatment, potassium ion buildup in the affected neurons could continue unchecked and eventually exceed 15 mM/L. Above this concentration, K^+ clearance from astrocyte spatial buffering would likely cease, causing accelerated K^+ flooding and more rapidly shrinking rest potentials. Eventually, these neurons would develop flattened voltages and reduced ability to form effective action potentials, causing a major reduction in activity. A severe decline in the impaired neurotransmitter's activity could dominate brain function and trigger the switch to depression.

The End of the Depression Phase: Mass-transport considerations indicate that a transition from depression back to mania should be expected and not a surprise. Severely disabled neurons experience greatly reduced K^+ ion outflow, while surviving clearance mechanisms continue to operate. This could gradually eliminate the $(K^+)_o$ flooding that had developed during mania, perhaps approaching 3 mM/L. Eventually, impaired brain sites could restore resting voltages and action potentials, signaling the end of bipolar's depression phase.

The Interval between Depression and the Return to Mania: Individuals with bipolar disorder typically enjoy a welcome period of relative wellness called euthymia, which occurs before the resumption of mania.[202,203] This delayed return to mania might result from medications or other treatments but has also been observed in many thousands of treatment-naïve patients. This temporary absence of troubling symptoms may involve two primary factors: (a) normalization of $(K^+)_o$ levels achieved during the depression phase, and (b) conformational and other adaptive changes in response to prolonged neuronal hyperactivity. For example, we know that voltage-gated Na^+ channels move farther from the hillock during periods of excessive activity, thus reducing the tendency for an action potential. In another example, postsynaptic receptors tend to develop reduced efficiency to compensate for prolonged excessive synaptic neurotransmitter levels. Although the resilience mechanisms are poorly known, it is expected that the propensity for neuronal hyperactivity is significantly reduced following weeks or months of mania and excessive neuronal firing. This would help explain the absence of mania immediately after the end of the depression phase. Patients with minimal adaptive changes may experience rapid cycling, whereas those with extensive adaptations may exhibit lengthy intervals before the return of mania.

The Return to Mania: After an extended period of reduced neuronal activity, the adaptive changes associated with mania's prolonged hyperactivity are likely to gradually fade away. Without effective treatment, the recovering brain will gradually return to mania but not normality, since the progressive ion channel damage that triggered bipolar disorder onset has not been repaired. Most treatment-naive bipolar patients report relatively mild symptoms as mania begins to return, followed by increasing severity and the tendency for another switch to temporary depression. Without effective treatment, a patient may be trapped in a lifetime of mania/depression cycles.

Switching Mechanism Discussion: It was exciting to identify a plausible mechanism for mania/depression switching, especially since the mechanism is consistent with the decisive role of ion channel and DNA-damage gene variants in bipolar disorder. As suspected, bipolar's depression phase may be caused by prolonged hyperactivity during mania. The GWAS data suggests that mania/depression switching is triggered by relentless additional DNA damage over time which temporarily disables a vulnerable neurotransmitter system. Numerous brain disorders including epilepsy, ADHD, anxiety/panic disorders, and phenotypes of schizophrenia involve prolonged neuronal hyperactivity without chronic switches to temporary depression. I believe that the unique difference in bipolar disorder is genetic and acquired impairments in the collaborative team of 400+ ion channel genes which increase vulnerability to neuronal instability.

This switching model involves an arbitrary assumption that the switch to depression is dominated by a single misbehaving neurotransmitter, and this may not be the case. In addition, it is important to note that bipolar onset might be caused by severe damage to an inhibitory neurotransmitter system such as serotonin or GABA that might delay the onset (or return) of mania. Also, there may be other switching mechanisms due to the multitude of possible combinations of damaged ion channels. In any case, this model assumes (a) the unstable transmitter's activity increases during bipolar disorder onset,

(b) becomes more hyperactive as potassium flooding progresses, and then (c) dramatically declines, causing the switch to depression. Since the switch involves unique severe poverty of a single neurotransmitter system, it appears likely that this mood disorder may not resemble other forms of clinical depression.

An important question to ask is as follows: Why could severe impairment be limited to a single neurotransmitter system, recognizing that the genetic and acquired weaknesses in ion channel genes and DNA repair capability would be shared by all parts of the brain? There are several plausible explanations for the heightened vulnerability of individual brain sites. For example, the protective blood-brain barrier is missing in certain limbic and brainstem areas. Also, epigenetic variations during development could impact neuronal activity or DNA integrity in individual cell types. In another example, some brain locations have relatively low astrocyte populations that assist $(K^+)_o$ clearance after neuron firing events. The next chapter describes a search for the impaired neurotransmitter system responsible for the switch to depression.

References

187. Pettigrew, J. D., & Miller, S. M. (1998). A 'sticky'interhemispheric switch in bipolar disorder?. *Proceedings of the Royal Society of London. Series B: Biological Sciences, 265*(1411), 2141–2148.
188. Grande, I., Bernardo, M., Bobes, J., Saiz-Ruiz, J., Álamo, C., & Vieta, E. (2014). Antipsychotic switching in bipolar disorders: a systematic review. *International Journal of Neuropsychopharmacology, 17*(3), 497–507.
189. Tamada, R. S., Issler, C. K., Amaral, J. A., Sachs, G. S., & Lafer, B. (2004). Treatment emergent affective switch: a controlled study. *Bipolar Disorders, 6*(4), 333–337.
190. Barnett, M. W., & Larkman, P. M. (2007). The action potential. *Practical neurology, 7*(3), 192–197.
191. Magioncalda, P., & Martino, M. (2022). A unified model of the pathophysiology of bipolar disorder. *Molecular Psychiatry, 27*(1), 202–211.
192. McGorry, P., Keshavan, M., Goldstone, S., Amminger, P., Allott, K., Berk, M., ... & Hickie, I. (2014). Biomarkers and clinical staging in psychiatry. *World Psychiatry, 13*(3), 211–223.

193. Berk, M., Dodd, S., Kauer-Sant'anna, M., Malhi, G. S., Bourin, M., Kapczinski, F., & Norman, T. (2007). Dopamine dysregulation syndrome: implications for a dopamine hypothesis of bipolar disorder. *Acta Psychiatrica Scandinavica, 116*, 41–49.

194. Rutecki, P. A. (1992). Neuronal excitability: voltage-dependent currents and synaptic transmission. *Journal of Clinical Neurophysiology, 9*(2), 195–211.

195. Murakami, S., & Kurachi, Y. (2016). Mechanisms of astrocytic K+ clearance and swelling under high extracellular K+ concentrations. *The journal of physiological sciences, 66*(2), 127–142.

196. Larsen, B. R., Stoica, A., & MacAulay, N. (2016). Managing brain extracellular K+ during neuronal activity: the physiological role of the Na+/K+-ATPase subunit isoforms. *Frontiers in physiology, 7*, 141.

197. Kofuji, P., & Connors, N. C. (2003). Molecular substrates of potassium spatial buffering in glial cells. *Molecular neurobiology, 28*, 195–208.

198. Chen, K. C., & Nicholson, C. (2000). Spatial buffering of potassium ions in brain extracellular space. *Biophysical journal, 78*(6), 2776–2797.

199. Lauritzen, M., Dreier, J. P., Fabricius, M., Hartings, J. A., Graf, R., & Strong, A. J. (2011). Clinical relevance of cortical spreading depression in neurological disorders: migraine, malignant stroke, subarachnoid and intracranial hemorrhage, and traumatic brain injury. *Journal of Cerebral Blood Flow & Metabolism, 31*(1), 17–35.

200. Cozzolino, O., Marchese, M., Trovato, F., Pracucci, E., Ratto, G. M., Buzzi, M. G., ... & Santorelli, F. M. (2018). Understanding spreading depression from headache to sudden unexpected death. *Frontiers in neurology, 9*, 19.

201. Gao, K., Lin, Z., Wen, S., & Jiang, Y. (2022). Potassium channels and epilepsy. *Acta Neurologica Scandinavica, 146*(6), 699–707.

202. Blumberg, H. P. (2012). Euthymia, depression, and mania: what do we know about the switch?. *Biological psychiatry, 71*(7), 10–1016.

203. Ozdel, O., Karadag, F., Atesci, F. C., Oguzhanoglu, N. K., & Cabuk, T. (2007). Cognitive functions in euthymic patients with bipolar disorder. *Annals of Saudi medicine, 27*(4), 273–278.

CHAPTER 10

A Search for the Switching Neurotransmitter

Introduction

The exclusion analysis of GWAS variants identified bipolar disorder as a channelopathy involving numerous mutated small-effect ion channel genes. This knowledge greatly narrowed the search for the switching mechanism that now focused exclusively on possible ion channel impairments. This activity resulted in identification of the mania/depression switching mechanism described in Chapter 9. According to this new model, bipolar onset begins when a genetically weakened ion channel team experiences additional DNA damage with age that alters neuronal activity of several neurotransmitters, resulting in mania. The switch to depression results from a severely damaged transmitter that develops extreme potassium ion flooding and shrinking rest voltages, causing a major decline in neuronal activity. An important feature of this model is an explanation for the return to mania and chronic mania/depression cycling in which the impaired transmitter recovers due to major reductions in potassium ion outflow while surviving clearance mechanisms continue to operate. Although this switching model is far from proven, it appears to be the most likely possibility based on today's information. Future advances in neuroscience will eventually resolve this uncertainty. At this stage of this investigation, there was little consensus regarding the identity of the misbehaving neurotransmitter with primary responsibility for bipolar disorder switching.

At this stage of this investigation, I was faced with an important question: If a single misbehaving NT is primarily responsible for bipolar switching, which one is it?

Neurotransmission Considerations

Interactive Neurotransmitters: For many years, dopamine, serotonin, norepinephrine, and other transmitters were regarded as somewhat isolated systems that acted independently. However, neuroscientists have learned that major neurotransmitters are intimately involved with each other and collaborate in many ways.[194,204] More than 140 receptor genes express unique receptors sensitive to a specific neurotransmitter that take up residence in membranes of diverse neurons throughout the brain. For example, a typical dopamine neuron has receptors for serotonin, GABA, glutamate, and other transmitters in its membranes. These foreign receptors have a major role in regulating the activity of every major neurotransmitter. Signaling of serotonin receptors embedded in dopamine membranes can effectively inhibit dopamine activity. In another example, signaling of norepinephrine receptors on serotonin neurons can have a major impact on serotonin activity. Significant progress in determining these interactive effects has been achieved in the past 25 years, but what we don't know still greatly exceeds what we have learned. A major complication is that foreign receptors have very different impacts at different transmitter sites. For example, serotonin has at least 14 receptor subtypes that may inhibit or enhance neuronal activity at other transmitters. Another complication is the impact of SNP mutations on receptors, MAO enzymes, reuptake transporters, etc. At present, the complexity of transmitter interactions is so great that one cannot predict the impact of a new treatment intervention with total confidence. It may take many years before a thorough understanding of collaborating neurotransmitter systems is achieved.

Challenges in Bipolar Disorder Research: Complex mechanisms of major neurotransmitters are now known in remarkable (although incomplete) detail, providing a valuable baseline for research. However, bipolar disorder presents unique challenges for experimental studies. Genetic ion channel impairments may alter permeabilities and gradients of Na^+, K^+, Ca^{++}, and Cl^- ions that may produce unfamiliar abnormal neuronal behavior. Prolonged hyperactivity during mania produces adaptive changes that may blur experimental results. As previously described, neurons respond to extreme hyperactivity by moving axon voltage-gated Na^+ ions further from the hillock.[205,206] In another example, abnormally high transmitter levels in synapses typically reduce the efficiency or population of postsynaptic receptors due to adaptive compensation.[207] There may be dozens of such adaptive responses during mania's prolonged hyperactivity episodes that researchers must cope with. Another challenge involves major changes in neurotransmission properties during different stages of mania and depression. Experimental studies during early mania or depression episodes may produce contradictory findings if repeated during late stages. Several recent studies have attempted to avoid this problem by testing patients during relatively stable euthymia intervals.[208]

Perhaps the greatest challenge involves studies of the severely impaired neurotransmitter responsible for switching.[209] Neuronal activity in the presence of excessive K^+ flooding may be dominated by shrinking potassium ion gradients and rest potentials, and not by reuptake, precursor levels, receptor efficiencies, and other factors that normally dominate neurotransmission. Hence, studies of a flooded transmitter's role in mania or depression may be prone to serious error. Experimenters introducing medications that inhibit reuptake might misinterpret a failure to increase manic activity. In another example, challenge experiments that alter transmitter concentrations in cytosol may have little impact if neuronal firing is dominated by shrinking rest potentials. In summary, experimental studies of an extremely dysregulated neurotransmitter system are prone to unreliable conclusions if they depend on typical responses to previously impactful factors.

Excitatory and Inhibitory Neurotransmitters: At bipolar onset, several transmitters may develop a stable degree of hyperactivity, with one of them experiencing out-of-control K^+ flooding. Norepinephrine, dopamine, and glutamate are excitatory, while GABA and serotonin generally have inhibitory effects on neuronal activity.[62] Any of these transmitters theoretically could cause a switch to depression if their neurons experienced severe potassium ion flooding. Gradual nonstop $(K^+)_o$ flooding at an excitatory transmitter could increase activity initially but develop poverty of action potentials as K^+ levels become excessive. In contrast, increasing hyperactivity of inhibitory neurons might initially reduce the activity of other transmitters, thereby delaying the appearance of mania, but it will eventually cause a loss of function due to the nonstop increases in $(K^+)_o$ levels. Regardless of inhibitory or excitatory properties, the bipolar switch to depression could be caused by declining activity in a neurotransmitter prominent in clinical depression.

Comparison of Switching Neurotransmitter Candidates

Over the past 30 years, the majority of thoughtful and evidence-based bipolar disorder theories placed primary blame on either dopamine, norepinephrine, or serotonin.[210,211,212] Other researchers have suggested major roles for glutamate or GABA. Each of these neurotransmitters could produce depression if activity sharply declined. The following analysis evaluated serotonin, dopamine, norepinephrine, glutamate, and GABA systems with respect to the relative likelihood of primary involvement in the switch from mania to depression.

My mania/depression switching model assumes especially severe ion channel damage to a vulnerable transmitter system that initially develops hyperactivity followed by a major decline in neurotransmissions. If this model is correct, researchers of bipolar disorder may have observed similar abnormal neuronal behavior in previous animal and human studies. Since oxidative overload and accelerated DNA damage are features of bipolar disorder, the neurotransmitter system responsible for switching may reside in a brain region with minimal blood-brain barrier protection. Also, this NT system would be expected to have a major role in sleep since sleeping difficulty is nearly universal in bipolar disorder patients. As discussed in Chapter 1, prolonged periods of severe mania and depression do not eliminate potential for high artistic, cognitive, or career capability since many present and historic individuals have achieved outstanding accomplishments despite severe bipolar depression. This suggests the misbehaving neurotransmitter may have relatively minor impacts on cognition. In addition, extremely low activity of most NT systems is associated with distinctive side effects that may or may not have been observed in prior bipolar research. The following pages examine each of the five suspect NT systems with respect to the following factors:

- Relative vulnerability to DNA damage,
- An important role in sleep,
- Retention of significant cognitive function,
- Evidence of very low activity during depression phases,
- Side effects associated with severely low activity.

Evaluation Criterion #1 - Relative Vulnerability to DNA Damage:
The brain is protected against physical damage by the skull, three
meninges, and cerebrospinal fluid that provides cushioning. However,
the primary protection against DNA damage is provided by the blood-
brain barrier (BBB), which was discovered accidentally by the great
Paul Ehrlich in the 1880s.[213,214] During an immunology experiment, he
injected blue dye into a mouse that permeated all tissues but unex-
pectedly was completely missing in the brain and spinal cord. A later
experiment showed that dyes injected into a mouse's brain failed to
reach the rest of its body (periphery). This led to the discovery that the
brain is biochemically isolated despite numerous blood vessels in the
brain that deliver nutrients to neurons and remove waste products.
After years of research, scientists learned that the interior surfaces
of the brain's blood vessels are covered by endothelial cells with
tight junctions that restrict the passage of toxins and other unwanted
chemicals.[215] This tight gap allows only small molecules, fat-soluble
molecules, and some gases to pass freely across capillary walls and
interact with neurons and glial cells. In addition, the BBB has a rich
array of ion channels and transporters that provide the brain with necessary biochemicals. A multitude of tiny blood capillaries perfuse the
entire brain, and most neurons are only 10–20 micrometers from a
blood vessel that delivers its supply of nutrients. The BBB provides
a defense against pathogens and toxins that may damage neurons,
while at the same time allowing glucose and other vital nutrients to
enter the brain.

　　While most of the brain enjoys good BBB protection, certain brainstem and limbic areas have minimal or zero protection. For example,
the pineal gland, pituitary, and parts of the third and fourth ventricle membranes are totally without BBB protection.[216] With respect
to DNA damage, the major offending substances from blood are (a)
toxic metals and other sources of free radical oxidative stress (ROS)
and inflammation and (b) chemicals that can form damaging adducts
that attach to DNA. The five NT systems under study exhibit significant differences in BBB protection. Glutamate and GABA molecules
originate in astrocytes scattered through the brain and enjoy relatively
good BBB protection. In contrast, norepinephrine originates at the
locus coeruleus (LC) in the upper brainstem, and there is evidence of
inflammation and unwanted substances in this region. The dopamine
system is primarily located in the substantia nigra, a part of the basal

ganglia near the third ventricle that has incomplete BBB protection. Serotonin is primarily synthesized in brainstem raphe nuclei that are near unprotected parts of the fourth ventricle. In addition, serotonin neurons in raphe nuclei are very susceptible to inflammation due to proximity to the cerebral aqueduct. Inflammation in the dorsal raphe brain location has been directly associated with manic-like behavior.[216] Based on published studies, the relative vulnerability of the five NT systems to DNA assault is summarized below

Relative Vulnerability to DNA Damage
- Serotonin: highest
- Norepinephrine: high
- Dopamine: high
- GABA: low
- Glutamate: low

Evaluation Criterion #2 - An Important Role in Sleep: More than 95% of our large bipolar disorder patient population reported serious sleep problems, especially during mania. Solid clinical progress rarely was achieved until a patient could get a good restful sleep. Some believe that effective sleep may be as essential to survival as food and water. Like an athlete's muscles after vigorous exercise, the brain may need a period of rest to recover from a day's strenuous activity. Scientists have learned that sleep plays a housekeeping role including removal of toxins and wastes, refueling with nutrients, and restoring the brain's supply of ATP (the molecule that provides energy to cells).[217,218] Sleep may also have a role in other important processes including consolidation of memories and normalizing ion gradients throughout the brain. Although not found in scientific literature, I believe sleep may also have a critical role in minimizing and repairing DNA damage. The brain's energy requirements while awake require high mitochondrial activity which is a major source of free radicals that assault DNA. It appears that wakefulness is a period of heightened DNA damage, and the quiescent hours during sleep may enhance repair of DNA that was assaulted during the day's activities. This might be analogous to giving your brain a "tune-up" every 24 hours.

The neuroscience of sleep is extremely complex, and each of the five NTs being evaluated has a significant role together with adenosine, histamine, and hypocretin (also called orexin).[219] The brain's hypothalamus is the key regulator of sleep and wakefulness, and its suprachiasmatic nuclei (SCN) serve as a "pacemaker" that regulates circadian timing. At any time, your brain will either be in a state of wakefulness, rapid eye movement (REM) sleep, or some stage of non-REM sleep. Serotonin, norepinephrine, glutamate, and dopamine neurons fire steadily during wakefulness, exhibit decreased activity during non-REM sleep, and may cease firing almost completely during REM sleep. GABA, produced in the hypothalamus, is primarily responsible for inhibition of neuronal firing during sleep. The brain exhibits significant activity during all phases of sleep, partly due to acetylcholine neurotransmissions. Adenosine gradually accumulates in extracellular spaces while we are awake, increasing sleeping pressure. Dopamine acts as a light sensor in the pineal gland and has a role in regulating sleep-inducing melatonin levels. Melatonin is synthesized from serotonin in the pineal gland, and dopamine levels increase during prolonged sleep absences. In summary, all five NT systems have important roles in sleep, with GABA perhaps exhibiting the greatest role. I conclude that sleep comparisons do not assist the search for the NT system responsible for bipolar disorder switching.

Evaluation Criterion #3 - Retention of Significant Cognitive Function: My clinical experience includes about 1,500 bipolar, 3,200 schizophrenia, 2,800 depression, and 1,400 anxiety patients. While most reported their illness seriously harmed their job or career, hundreds were still leaders in their field with quite remarkable accomplishments. My clinical population included captains of industry, billionaires, scientists, medical doctors, Academy Award winners, Olympic Games champions, NBA players, professional golfers, a world heavyweight champion, a Miss America winner, and two symphony conductors. I learned firsthand that fame and fortune do not guarantee happiness. I also learned that a very large percentage of high achievers in my clinical population were diagnosed with bipolar disorder. This is not a surprise since Churchill, Newton, Van Gogh, Dickens, Hemingway, and other historical figures displayed impressive cognition despite a severe version of the illness. While many of our bipolar achievers excelled during hypomania episodes, others spoke of doing their best work while in the depths of suicidal depression. Several achievers reported obsessive-compulsive tendencies and perfectionism that may have driven them to excel despite the illness. It seems likely that the NT system responsible for the depression switch would have relatively little impact on the prefrontal cortex (PFC) and other major cognition sites despite extraordinary reductions in this transmitter's activity for prolonged periods. The five candidate NT systems are here compared with respect to their role in learning and intellectual activities and the relative impact of hypothetical extreme reductions in neurotransmission during the depression phase.

> *Glutamate and GABA*: Glutamate is the brain's most prolific NT system and is responsible for about 90% of excitatory neurotransmissions. It is a precursor for the synthesis of GABA, which is the brain's primary inhibitory NT that helps regulate glutamate activity. Healthy brain function requires a good balance between glutamate and GABA. With respect to cognition, depressed glutamate activity has been associated with major deficits in learning and memory, as well as implicated in ADHD.[220] Similarly, the GABA system has a major role in most aspects of cognition, including interneuron functioning and memory processing in the entorhinal cortex and hippocampus. Low GABA activity has been associated with ADHD and other learning disorders. Both glutamate and GABA are intimately involved in all aspects of cognition. However, this bipolar disorder model involves a lengthy massive decline in activity of the neurotransmitter responsible for the switch to depression. Since collaborating glutamate and GABA systems are involved in 80–90% of all brain activity, it seems unlikely that a person could retain excellent cognitive capability if either system were severely impaired for an extended period.

> *Dopamine, Norepinephrine, and Serotonin*: As described by Stahl and others, efferent dopamine and norepinephrine neurons have major projections to the prefrontal cortex and other major cognition centers, whereas serotonin does not.[25] There is abundant evidence of dopamine's major roles in intellectual capacity and executive function.[221,222] For example, ADHD is associated with depressed dopamine activity. For decades, Ritalin, Adderall, and other dopaminergic medications have exhibited impressive efficacy at focusing attention. In another example, numerous studies report cognitive deficits in Parkinson's patients following significant loss of dopamine neurons. Dopamine has a major role in learning, working memory, and

decision-making in the prefrontal cortex. A dramatic loss in dopamine activity during bipolar's depression phase appears inconsistent with cognitive excellence. Efferent norepinephrine neurons also project to the PFC and have a major role in working memory, attention, planning, and other cognitive functions.[223] Some neuroscientists believe norepinephrine is the primary modulator and regulator of the PFC, and there is strong evidence that suppressed norepinephrine activity can impair the PFC and cognitive capability. This suggests blunted intellectual ability would result from severe norepinephrine hypoactivity during the depression phase. Compared to dopamine and norepinephrine, fewer serotonin (5-HT) neurons project to major cognition centers, and depressed serotonin levels are believed to have a less impactful influence on intelligence and executive function. In summary, while serotonin has significant roles in memory processing and other executive functions, this analysis indicates it has far less effect on cognition than the other NT switching candidates.

Evaluation Criterion #4 - Evidence of Very Low Activity during Depression Phases:

A neuron's activity represents the rate at which its transmitters are ejected into a synapse.[62] Neurotransmission (also called signaling) requires interaction with a nearby postsynaptic receptor. Each neurotransmitter's axons project to numerous brain sites and spray their unique transmitters into local synapses. Receptors are specialized genetically expressed ion channels imbedded in neuronal membranes that generally can be activated only by a single transmitter type (serotonin, dopamine, etc.). Each of the five candidate NT systems has a full spectrum of receptors for foreign transmitters on their neuronal membranes that affect their behavior. About 140 unique receptor subtypes may or may not take up residency at each of our 80 billion brain neurons. This helps explain the great complexity of NT interactions.

Dopamine: Over the past 20 years, dopamine theories of bipolar disorder have begun to dominate the attention of many neuroscientists.[193,210] Dopamine hyperactivity is a dominant feature of bipolar's mania phase, and dopamine hypoactivity is associated with forms of clinical depression. This has led dopamine researchers to seek plausible neuroscience mechanisms that may explain chronic switching between mania and depression. Numerous experimental studies have consistently reported elevated dopamine activity during mania. Moreover, medications that reduce dopamine activity have demonstrated efficacy in combating mania and have become mainstream therapies. Molecular imaging and pharmacological studies suggest that increased D_2 and D_3 receptor availability and associated dopamine hyperactivity may be essential features of mania. Other studies report prefrontal D_1 receptors mediate anxiety, reward, memory, and inflammation that are associated with bipolar disorder. Elevated dopamine activity has also been associated with anxiety, hyperactivity, mood swings, sleep disorders, and psychosis. It's clear that dopamine neurons are very hyperactive during bipolar disorder's manic phase. However, the role of dopamine during the depression phase is far less clear. Especially puzzling are contradictory experimental studies that indicate significant efficacy from either increasing or decreasing dopamine activity during bipolar's depression periods. Three double-blind, placebo-controlled studies reported efficacy from medication enhancement of D_2/D_3 receptors during depression episodes.[210] However, other studies report that Zyprexa and other dopamine antagonists are beneficial during the depression phase. This paradox is still unresolved, and dopamine's behavior during bipolar's depression phase remains uncertain. I believe this disparity might be related to major changes in neuronal activity as impaired neurons recover. Additional research will be necessary to determine if major dopamine hypoactivity is a feature of bipolar's depression episodes. In my opinion, the double-blind D_2/D_3 studies are more convincing. For example, 2nd generation atypical medications exhibit antioxidant properties and may provide benefits unrelated to dopamine activity.[224,225] In summary, it is very likely (but not proven) that dopamine is hypoactive during bipolar's depression phase.

Norepinephrine: This neurotransmitter has been associated with bipolar disorder for more than 50 years, and norepinephrine theories of bipolar disorder continue to attract attention.[212] Also known as noradrenaline, norepinephrine is formed in the brain's locus coeruleus by the addition of a hydroxyl group to a dopamine molecule. Although very small in number, these neurons increase alertness, arousal, and attention and have a major cognitive role in the prefrontal cortex. In addition, this versatile transmitter impacts mood, memory, the sleep-wake cycle, regulation of blood pressure, protection against inflammation, and several other important functions. Elevated norepinephrine activity is a classic feature of bipolar's manic phase, and most manic and hypomanic patients benefit from medications that antagonize this neurotransmitter system. In addition, low norepinephrine activity is associated with clinical depression which suggests a possible major role in bipolar disorder switching.[225] During the depression phase, SNRI medications that increase both serotonin and norepinephrine activity are more effective than serotonin-enhancing SSRI medications alone.[226,227] This is consistent with low norepinephrine activity after the switch to depression. In summary, norepinephrine exhibits major hyperactivity during mania, and there is considerable evidence of hypoactivity during bipolar's depression phase.

Glutamate: Several studies indicate depressed glutamate activity in major depression disorder (MDD).[228] In addition, depressed glutamate activity has been associated with low energy, anxiety, and insomnia, which are features of bipolar's depression episodes. There is little doubt that depressed glutamate activity could result in clinical depression. However, research studies have consistently indicated elevated glutamate activity throughout bipolar disorder phases.[229,230] Ketamine, N-acetylcysteine (NAC), lamotrigine, and other glutamate inhibitors have displayed efficacy during bipolar's depression phase episodes.[231] In addition, experimental evidence of elevated glutamate/glutamine ratios during bipolar depression suggests hyperactivity.[232] In summary, several studies indicate that glutamate neurons are not hypoactive during bipolar's depression phase.

GABA: There is limited reliable evidence of GABA's role during bipolar's depression phase.[233,234] Numerous experimental studies have produced conflicting results, reporting either elevated or depressed GABA activity. Magnetic resonance spectroscopy (MRS) of stably medicated euthymia patients indicated higher GABA levels at two brain cortex sites, compared to healthy controls. Several plasma studies (which have limited validity regarding brain behavior) have indicated low GABA levels during bipolar's depression and euthymia phases, while other plasma studies have reported GABA elevations. Cerebrospinal fluid studies have also failed to consistently indicate elevated or depressed GABA levels. Most studies have involved patients who were taking medications that are known to impact GABA activity. In summary, despite dozens of careful studies, there is no solid evidence of low GABA activity during bipolar disorder's depression phase, and there is certainly no evidence of a severe poverty of GABA action potentials.

Serotonin: Over the past 50 years, experimental studies have consistently reported low serotonin activity during bipolar's depression phase.[235,236] In addition, serotonin-enhancement therapies have generally indicated some degree of efficacy during bipolar's depression episodes. However, these clinical improvements are usually disappointing compared to typical effectiveness of SSRI medications in treatment of unipolar depression. In addition, SSRI antidepressants occasionally trigger sudden mania, causing many clinicians to reduce or eliminate use of antidepressants for bipolar patients.[237,238] Plasma and whole blood testing of our large bipolar population indicated 5–10% were overmethylated and we learned this group has a high incidence of SSRI intolerance. This is not surprising because epigenetic research indicates that differences in global DNA methyl content have a major impact on neurotransmissions and depression.[239] This suggests that mania risk from use of antidepressants may result more directly from altered methylation at histones and DNA's CpG islands and not higher serotonin activity. In summary, I conclude there is clear evidence of depressed serotonin activity during bipolar disorder's depression phase.

The above comparative analysis was limited by a lack of decisive experimental evidence of neurotransmission rates during bipolar's depression phase. Based on the available information, the relative certitude of low activity during the depression phase for the five candidate NT systems is summarized below:

- Serotonin: Definite hypoactivity.
- Norepinephrine: Strong evidence of hypoactivity.
- Dopamine: Likely hypoactive (but not 100% certain).
- GABA: No strong evidence of hypoactivity.
- Glutamate: Current evidence suggests **hyper**activity.

Evaluation Criterion #5 – Side Effects Associated with Severely Low Activity: The switching model describes a neurotransmitter system that is significantly disabled for an extended period after the switch to depression. Prior research has identified typical behaviors and other side effects associated with very low neuronal activity for several neurotransmitters. The glutamate, GABA, dopamine, nor-epinephrine, and serotonin systems were examined for presence or absence of symptoms/behaviors associated with very low activity.

> *Glutamate*: Very depressed glutamate activity at NMDA receptors has been associated with a major schizophrenia phenotype,[240] and more than 50% of patients diagnosed with bipolar disorder develop psychotic symptoms during their lifetimes.[241] This low-glutamate schizophrenia phenotype presents as a high dopamine sensory disorder with auditory hallucinations as a dominant symptom. However, the great majority of our 600+ bipolar-diagnosed patients with a history of psychosis exhibited severe delusions associated with excessive glutamate activity at NMDA receptors. This population also had a high incidence of OCD behaviors and undermethylation that are associated with excessive glutamate activity.[36] Extremely low glutamate activity has been associated with very low blood pressure and functional movement disorders, and these are not commonly found in unmedicated bipolar patients.[242] In summary, clear evidence of behaviors or side effects associated with depressed glutamate activity during bipolar's depression phase were not observed. This is not surprising because there is considerable evidence that glutamate activity is elevated and not depressed during bipolar's depression phase.

> *GABA*: Symptoms of low GABA activity in adults include lethargy, EEG abnormalities, seizure tendencies, psychomotor retardation (PR), insomnia, and anxiety.[243,244,245] Lethargy, insomnia, and anxiety are common features of bipolar's depression phase. Psychomotor retardation typically involves self-touching behaviors and slow movements of hands, legs, and torso. While self-touching is not a feature of bipolar's depression episodes, slow leg, hand, and torso movements are consistent with general lethargy. Increased seizure risk has been associated with mania but not during bipolar's depression phase. In summary, while several low GABA behaviors have been observed,

the absence of elevated seizure activity suggests that GABA activity is not severely depressed during bipolar's depression phase.

Dopamine: Dopamine is a "feel-good" neurotransmitter associated with pleasure, a positive attitude, and motivation. Many studies report that low dopamine levels are associated with anhedonia, which is a psychiatric term for inability to experience pleasure.[246] Anhedonia is a common feature of bipolar's depression phase and has been implicated in this disorder's high suicide risk. This is consistent with low dopamine activity in bipolar depression. However, a contrary finding involves absence of serious extrapyramidal symptoms (EPS) (shaking and other abnormal movements) during bipolar's depression episodes. There is abundant evidence that extended and severely depressed dopamine activity is associated with major movement symptoms.[247] While bipolar disorder involves a slight increased risk for Parkinson's disease, significant movement disorders are not a typical feature of the depression phase.[248,249] In Parkinson's disease, progressive death of dopamine cells (apoptosis) typically results in uncontrollable shaking. In addition, schizophrenia medications that lower dopamine activity are plagued by tardive dyskinesia, a common movement side effect that often becomes permanent.[250] These somewhat conflicting results might be explained by mild-to-moderate hypoactivity associated with depression, ADHD, and anhedonia that lacks severity needed for extrapyramidal movements. In summary, several low dopamine behaviors have been observed during bipolar's depression phase, but the absence of major extrapyramidal movements is inconsistent with prolonged very low dopamine activity.

Norepinephrine: Depressed norepinephrine activity has been associated with fibromyalgia and chronic fatigue which are frequent features of bipolar's depression phase.[251,252] In the brain, this neurotransmitter has many functions, including regulation of blood pressure. While high norepinephrine activity is associated with hypertension, low activity is associated with low blood pressure levels.[253] Dopamine beta-hydroxylase (DBH) deficiency syndrome involves greatly reduced norepinephrine activity and is characterized by extremely low blood pressure levels.[254] Norepinephrine infusions are a first-line emergency treatment for severe low blood pressure.[255] Several experimental studies have reported reduced blood pressure during bipolar's depression episodes, and this is consistent with norepinephrine hypoactivity after the switch to depression. However, these blood pressure levels were generally minor rather than severely low. A recent study reported that modest reductions in norepinephrine activity have little or no impact on blood pressure. In summary, fibromyalgia, chronic fatigue, and reduced blood pressure provide supporting evidence of norepinephrine hypoactivity during bipolar's depression phase, but the slight blood pressure drop suggests the activity decrement may not be severe.

Serotonin: Nearly all the brain's serotonin is produced in the raphe nuclei located in the center of the brainstem. Raphe nuclei include nine separate layers of serotonin neurons that have very different functions. Three caudal layers descend into the spinal cord and influence pain regulation, blood clotting, and other body functions. Bipolar disorder studies generally report increased pain sensation (which means lower pain threshold) compared to controls.[256] Blood clotting is also prevalent in bipolar patients, but this may be related to medication side effects. Dorsal, medial, and other rostral neurons ascend into the midbrain, cortex, and other brain sites and spray serotonin into synapses throughout much of the brain. The number one symptom of serotonin hypoactivity is depression. Other low serotonin associations include OCD, impulsivity, aggression, anhedonia, insomnia, and high suicide risk.[257,258,259] Each of these comorbidities has been found at an increased incidence in bipolar disorder studies and are major features of bipolar disorder's depression phase. A 2018 mouse study reported extremely low serotonin activity produced abnormal behavior that closely resembled mania in bipolar patients.[260] All of these factors neatly fit the new bipolar model that posits a major decline in the dysregulated transmitter's activity after the switch to depression. In summary, most classic symptoms of serotonin hypoactivity are features of bipolar disorder's depression phase.

This evaluation (#5) examined the presence or absence of behaviors and side-effects expected in the event of severe hypoactivity for each of the five candidate neurotransmitters. Significant inconsistencies associated with prolonged low activity are summarized below:

- Serotonin: None.
- Norepinephrine: Absence of a major decline in blood pressure.
- GABA: Absence of major seizures.
- Dopamine: Absence of major extrapyramidal symptoms (shaking, etc.).
- Glutamate: Evidence points to **hyper**activity, not **hypo**activity.

Switching Neurotransmitter Investigation Results

In this chapter, the five candidate neurotransmitter systems were evaluated with respect to vulnerability to DNA damage, role in sleep, impact on cognition, evidence of major hypoactivity during bipolar's depression phase, and side-effects associated with severe hypoactivity. This analysis compares the compatibility of each transmitter with the new switching model that assumes continuous $(K^+)_o$ flooding at a vulnerable transmitter's neurons, resulting in initial hyperactivity followed by temporary major hypoactivity. Figure 17 summarizes the results of this analysis that points to serotonin as the dysregulated transmitter responsible for the switch to depression. This was a surprise since dozens of research studies have suggested that dopamine and norepinephrine exhibit more dominant roles in bipolar disorder.

	Dopamine	Norepinephrine	Serotonin	GABA	Glutamate
Vulnerability to DNA Damage	✓	✓	✓	✗	✗
Importance in Sleep	✓	✓	✓	✓	✓
Retention of Cognitive Function	✗	✗	✓	✗	✗
Hypoactivity During Depression Stage	✓	✓	✓	✗	✗
Presence of Expected Side Effects from Hypoactivity	✗	✗	✓	✓ / ✗	✗

Figure 17. Compatibility with the Advanced Bipolar Disorder Model

An impaired serotonin system is very consistent with the new bipolar disorder model, whereas the other candidate neurotransmitter systems exhibit definite areas of incompatibility. Factors in support of a dominant role for serotonin in switching include (a) relatively high vulnerability to DNA damage and inflammation, (b) a major role in sleep, (c) limited blunting of cognition during major hypoactivity, (d) high frequency of OCD, aggression, anhedonia, suicide, and other hypoactivity symptoms, and (e) depression phase studies indicate low serotonin activity and reduced depression severity following activity-enhancement interventions. The dopamine and norepinephrine systems each exhibit hyperactivity at mania onset, and there is evidence that both exhibit hypoactivity during the depression phase. However, these activity declines appear modest compared to the major impairments described in the new bipolar disorder model. In addition, dopamine and norepinephrine are major contributors to cognition, which appears inconsistent with the remarkable accomplishments of numerous people during the throes of severe bipolar depression. Major declines in dopamine activity are associated with shaking and other movement abnormalities that are typically absent during bipolar disorder's depression phase. Also, major reductions in blood pressure associated with very depressed norepinephrine activity have not been reported. The GABA and glutamate systems are relatively well protected by the blood-brain barrier and may be less vulnerable to DNA damage. Both systems have significant cognition roles that are somewhat inconsistent with occasional great accomplishments achieved during severe bipolar depression. Some studies have reported elevated GABA activity during the depression phase, while others have found depressed activity. It seems clear that the GABA system does not exhibit the major activity decline associated with the switching model. In addition, increased seizures associated with low GABA activity have not been reported. The glutamate system seems completely incompatible with the switching model since there is strong evidence of high activity during the depression phase.

The dominance of serotonin in bipolar switching appears highly likely based on this analysis, but it is not 100% proven. This finding depends on the validity of the new bipolar disorder model. In addition, this analysis is based on an arbitrary exclusion of acetylcholine, histamine, and other neurotransmitter systems that may have important roles in mania/depression transitions.

With these caveats and absence of 100% certainty, I conclude that an impaired and dysregulated serotonin system is responsible for the mania/depression switch in bipolar disorder.

References

204. Hyman, S. E. (2005). Neurotransmitters. *Current biology, 15*(5), R154-R158.
205. Grubb, M. S., & Burrone, J. (2010). Activity-dependent relocation of the axon initial segment fine-tunes neuronal excitability. *Nature, 465*(7301), 1070–1074.
206. Grubb, M. S., Shu, Y., Kuba, H., Rasband, M. N., Wimmer, V. C., & Bender, K. J. (2011). Short-and long-term plasticity at the axon initial segment. *Journal of Neuroscience, 31*(45), 16049–16055.
207. Cotovio, G., & Oliveira-Maia, A. J. (2022). Functional neuroanatomy of mania. *Translational Psychiatry, 12*(1), 29.
208. Singh, A., Pandey, H. R., Arya, A., Agarwal, V., Shree, R., & Kumar, U. (2023). Altered white matter integrity in euthymic children with bipolar disorder: a tract-based spatial statistical analysis of diffusion tensor imaging. *Journal of Affective Disorders, 340*, 820–827.
209. Young, J. W., & Dulcis, D. (2015). Investigating the mechanism (s) underlying switching between states in bipolar disorder. *European journal of pharmacology, 759*, 151–162.
210. Ashok, A. H., Marques, T. R., Jauhar, S., Nour, M. M., Goodwin, G. M., Young, A. H., & Howes, O. D. (2017). The dopamine hypothesis of bipolar affective disorder: the state of the art and implications for treatment. *Molecular psychiatry, 22*(5), 666–679.
211. Moncrieff, J., Cooper, R. E., Stockmann, T., Amendola, S., Hengartner, M. P., & Horowitz, M. A. (2023). The serotonin theory of depression: a systematic umbrella review of the evidence. *Molecular psychiatry, 28*(8), 3243–3256.
212. Kurita, M. (2016). Noradrenaline plays a critical role in the switch to a manic episode and treatment of a depressive episode. *Neuropsychiatric disease and treatment*, 2373–2380.
213. Daneman, R., & Prat, A. (2015). The blood–brain barrier. *Cold Spring Harbor perspectives in biology, 7*(1), a020412.
214. Dyrna, F., Hanske, S., Krueger, M., & Bechmann, I. (2013). The blood-brain barrier. *Journal of Neuroimmune Pharmacology, 8*, 763–773.

215. Wu, D., Chen, Q., Chen, X., Han, F., Chen, Z., & Wang, Y. (2023). The blood–brain barrier: Structure, regulation and drug delivery. *Signal transduction and targeted therapy, 8*(1), 217.

216. Maddaloni, G., Migliarini, S., Napolitano, F., Giorgi, A., Nazzi, S., Biasci, D., ... & Pasqualetti, M. (2018). Serotonin depletion causes valproate-responsive manic-like condition and increased hippocampal neuroplasticity that are reversed by stress. *Scientific Reports, 8*(1), 11847.

217. Hobson, J. A., & Pace-Schott, E. F. (2002). The cognitive neuroscience of sleep: neuronal systems, consciousness and learning. *Nature Reviews Neuroscience, 3*(9), 679–693.

218. Saper, C. B., Scammell, T. E., & Lu, J. (2005). Hypothalamic regulation of sleep and circadian rhythms. *Nature, 437*(7063), 1257–1263.

219. Schwartz, M. D., & Kilduff, T. S. (2015). The neurobiology of sleep and wakefulness. *The Psychiatric Clinics of North America, 38*(4), 615.

220. Reddy-Thootkur, M., Kraguljac, N. V., & Lahti, A. C. (2022). The role of glutamate and GABA in cognitive dysfunction in schizophrenia and mood disorders–A systematic review of magnetic resonance spectroscopy studies. *Schizophrenia research, 249*, 74–84.

221. Swanson, J. M., Flodman, P., Kennedy, J., Spence, M. A., Moyzis, R., Schuck, S., ... & Posner, M. (2000). Dopamine genes and ADHD. *Neuroscience & Biobehavioral Reviews, 24*(1), 21–25.

222. Wu, J., Xiao, H., Sun, H., Zou, L., & Zhu, L. Q. (2012). Role of dopamine receptors in ADHD: a systematic meta-analysis. *Molecular neurobiology, 45*(3), 605–620.

223. Holland, N., Robbins, T. W., & Rowe, J. B. (2021). The role of noradrenaline in cognition and cognitive disorders. *Brain, 144*(8), 2243–2256.

224. Aliyazicioglu, R., Kural, B., Çolak, M., Karahan, S. C., Ayvaz, S., & Deger, O. (2007). Treatment with lithium, alone or in combination with olanzapine, relieves oxidative stress but increases atherogenic lipids in bipolar disorder. *The Tohoku journal of experimental medicine, 213*(1), 79–87.

225. Dietrich-Muszalska, A., Kolodziejczyk-Czepas, J., & Nowak, P. (2021). Comparative study of the effects of atypical antipsychotic drugs on plasma and urine biomarkers of oxidative stress in schizophrenic patients. *Neuropsychiatric disease and treatment*, 555–565.

226. Palaniyappan, L., Insole, L., & Ferrier, N. (2009). Combining antidepressants: a review of evidence. *Advances in psychiatric treatment, 15*(2), 90–99.

227. Gitlin, M. J. (2018). Antidepressants in bipolar depression: an enduring controversy. *International journal of bipolar disorders, 6*(1), 25.

228. Khoodoruth, M. A. S., Estudillo-Guerra, M. A., Pacheco-Barrios, K., Nyundo, A., Chapa-Koloffon, G., & Ouanes, S. (2022). Glutamatergic system in depression and its role in neuromodulatory techniques optimization. *Frontiers in Psychiatry, 13*, 886918.

229. Hashimoto, K., Sawa, A., & Iyo, M. (2007). Increased levels of glutamate in brains from patients with mood disorders. *Biological psychiatry, 62*(11), 1310–1316.

230. Shen, J., & Tomar, J. S. (2021). Elevated brain glutamate levels in bipolar disorder and pyruvate carboxylase-mediated anaplerosis. *Frontiers in Psychiatry, 12*, 640977.

231. Bennett, R., Yavorsky, C., & Bravo, G. (2022). Ketamine for bipolar depression: Biochemical, psychotherapeutic, and psychedelic approaches. *Frontiers in Psychiatry, 13*, 867484.

232. Chen, G., Henter, I. D., & Manji, H. K. (2010). Presynaptic glutamatergic dysfunction in bipolar disorder. *Biological psychiatry, 67*(11), 1007.

233. Brady Jr, R. O., McCarthy, J. M., Prescot, A. P., Jensen, J. E., Cooper, A. J., Cohen, B. M., ... & Öngür, D. (2013). Brain gamma-aminobutyric acid (GABA) abnormalities in bipolar disorder. *Bipolar disorders, 15*(4), 434–439.

234. Kaufman, R. E., Ostacher, M. J., Marks, E. H., Simon, N. M., Sachs, G. S., Jensen, J. E., ... & Pollack, M. H. (2009). Brain GABA levels in patients with bipolar disorder. *Progress in Neuro-Psychopharmacology and Biological Psychiatry, 33*(3), 427–434.

235. Mahmood, T., & Silverstone, T. (2001). Serotonin and bipolar disorder. *Journal of affective disorders, 66*(1), 1–11.

236. Lan, M. J., & Mann, J. J. (2016). Serotonergic dysfunction in bipolar disorder. *Bipolar Disorders: Basic Mechanisms and Therapeutic Implications*, 43.

237. Tondo, L., Vázquez, G., & Baldessarini, R. J. (2010). Mania associated with antidepressant treatment: comprehensive meta-analytic review. *Acta Psychiatrica Scandinavica, 121*(6), 404–414.

238. Chun, B. J., & Dunner, D. L. (2004). A review of antidepressant-induced hypomania in major depression: suggestions for DSM-V. *Bipolar disorders, 6*(1), 32–42.

239. Chen, D., Meng, L., Pei, F., Zheng, Y., & Leng, J. (2017). A review of DNA methylation in depression. *Journal of Clinical Neuroscience, 43*, 39–46.

240. Uno, Y., & Coyle, J. T. (2019). Glutamate hypothesis in schizophrenia. *Psychiatry and clinical neurosciences, 73*(5), 204–215.

241. Kruse, A. O., & Bustillo, J. R. (2022). Glutamatergic dysfunction in Schizophrenia. *Translational Psychiatry, 12*(1), 500.

242. Westhoff, T. H., Schubert, F., Wirth, C., Joppke, M., Klär, A. A., Zidek, W., & Gallinat, J. (2011). The impact of blood pressure on hippocampal glutamate and mnestic function. *Journal of human hypertension, 25*(4), 256–261.

243. Ting Wong, C. G., Bottiglieri, T., & Snead III, O. C. (2003). Gaba, γ-hydroxybutyric acid, and neurological disease. *Annals of Neurology: Official Journal of the American Neurological Association and the Child Neurology Society, 54*(S6), S3-S12.

244. Cocchi, R. (1978). A syndrome from a possible GABA deficiency. Clinical-therapeutic report on 15 cases. *Acta Psychiatrica Belgica, 78*(2), 407–424.

245. Hepsomali, P., Groeger, J. A., Nishihira, J., & Scholey, A. (2020). Effects of oral gamma-aminobutyric acid (GABA) administration on stress and sleep in humans: A systematic review. *Frontiers in neuroscience, 14*, 559962.

246. Wise, R. A. (2008). Dopamine and reward: the anhedonia hypothesis 30 years on. *Neurotoxicity research, 14*(2), 169–183.

247. Sykes, D. A., Moore, H., Stott, L., Holliday, N., Javitch, J. A., Lane, J. R., & Charlton, S. J. (2017). Extrapyramidal side effects of antipsychotics are linked to their association kinetics at dopamine D2 receptors. *Nature communications, 8*(1), 763.

248. Dols, A., & Lemstra, A. W. (2020). Parkinsonism and bipolar disorder. *Bipolar Disorders, 22*(4), 413.

249. Faustino, P. R., Duarte, G. S., Chendo, I., Caldas, A. C., Reimão, S., Fernandes, R. M., ... & Ferreira, J. J. (2020). Risk of developing Parkinson disease in bipolar disorder: a systematic review and meta-analysis. *JAMA neurology, 77*(2), 192–198.

250. Carbon, M., Hsieh, C. H., Kane, J. M., & Correll, C. U. (2017). Tardive dyskinesia prevalence in the period of second-generation antipsychotic use: a meta-analysis. *The Journal of clinical psychiatry, 78*(3), 20738.

251. Mease, P. J. (2009). Further strategies for treating fibromyalgia: the role of serotonin and norepinephrine reuptake inhibitors. *The American journal of medicine, 122*(12), S44-S55.

252. Wyller, V. B., Vitelli, V., Sulheim, D., Fagermoen, E., Winger, A., Godang, K., & Bollerslev, J. (2016). Altered neuroendocrine control and association to clinical symptoms in adolescent chronic fatigue syndrome: a cross-sectional study. *Journal of Translational Medicine, 14*, 1–12.

253. Ungerleider, R. M., McMillan, K. N., Cooper, D. S., Meliones, J. N., & Jacobs, J. (2018). *Critical Heart Disease in Infants and Children E-Book: Critical Heart Disease in Infants and Children E-Book.* Elsevier Health Sciences.

254. Palma, J.-A., Norcliffe-Kaufmann, L., Fuente-Mora, C., Percival, L., Spalink, C. L., & Kaufmann, H. (2018). Disorders of the Autonomic Nervous System: Autonomic Dysfunction in Pediatric Practice. In *Swaiman's Pediatric Neurology* (6th ed., pp. 1173–1183). Elsevier.

255. Girbes, A. R. J., & Hoogenberg, K. (1998). The use of dopamine and norepinephrine in the ICU. *Yearbook of Intensive Care and Emergency Medicine 1998*, 178–187.

256. Zhao, H. Q., Zhou, M., Jiang, J. Q., Luo, Z. Q., & Wang, Y. H. (2024). Global trends and hotspots in pain associated with bipolar disorder in the last 20 years: a bibliometric analysis. *Frontiers in Neurology, 15*, 1393022.

257. Westenberg, H. G., Fineberg, N. A., & Denys, D. (2007). Neurobiology of obsessive-compulsive disorder: serotonin and beyond. *CNS spectrums, 12*(S3), 14–27.

258. Der-Avakian, A., & Markou, A. (2012). The neurobiology of anhedonia and other reward-related deficits. *Trends in neurosciences, 35*(1), 68–77.

259. Seo, D., Patrick, C. J., & Kennealy, P. J. (2008). Role of serotonin and dopamine system interactions in the neurobiology of impulsive aggression and its comorbidity with other clinical disorders. *Aggression and violent behavior, 13*(5), 383–395.

260. Shiah, I. S., & Yatham, L. N. (2000). Serotonin in mania and in the mechanism of action of mood stabilizers: a review of clinical studies. *Bipolar Disorders, 2*(2), 77–92.

CHAPTER 11

The Essence of Bipolar Disorder

After more than a century of mystery and uncertainty, the true nature of bipolar disorder is coming into view. The world's 250,000+ neuroscientists have achieved remarkable advances in understanding the extraordinary complexity of healthy brain function and have identified a multitude of distinctive differences associated with bipolar disorder. Guided by this information and recent GWAS research, this multiyear investigation may have resolved important unknowns that have puzzled scientists for more than a century.

The Cause of Bipolar Disorder

The exclusion analysis of bipolar variants indicates that coincident (a) ion channel mutations and (b) accelerated DNA damage dominate the genetic predisposition for bipolar disorder. Genetic weakness in the collaborative team of 400+ ion channels explains the vulnerability for impaired regulation of NTs and the onset of mania. The discovery that accelerated DNA damage is a prerequisite for the disorder is confirmed by dozens of published studies that report severe oxidative overload in bipolar patients. The remarkable stability of NTs and action potentials is gradually eroded by many years of progressive DNA damage to neurons and other brain sites. These mutations usually are not sufficient to trigger bipolar disorder during childhood and adolescence, but continuing DNA damage over many years eventually triggers bipolar onset.

Accelerated DNA Damage: All DNA molecules experience some degree of unrepaired damage every day, and this is why we age and are prone to future physical and mental disorders. Our antioxidant and DNA-repair genes protect against abnormal rates of damage, but research studies consistently report elevated oxidative stress and inadequate DNA-repair mechanisms in bipolar disorder. The exclusion analysis in Chapter 8 discovered that 75% of known pro-bipolar variants are prominent cancer and other DNA-damage genes. In addition, recent cancer research[261,262] indicates that impaired ion channels are associated with significant DNA damage. This includes specific mechanisms and impacts of mutated Na^+, K^+, Ca^{++}, and Cl^- ion channel genes that weaken DNA-damage response.[263,264,265,266,267] As a channelopathy, bipolar disorder experiences this additional source of oxidative stress that contributes to accelerated DNA damage. Relentless DNA damage continues after bipolar disorder onset, causing progressive severity and complexity of the illness. Hundreds of our bipolar disorder patients complained that medications that were quite effective in their 20s were no longer effective. In addition, excessive DNA damage rates are associated with oxidative overload and brain inflammation, which can aggravate symptoms.

Mania/Depression Switching Mechanism: The realization that bipolar disorder is a channelopathy led to an exhaustive search for ion channel impairments that might cause switching. Several hypothetical ion channel abnormalities were found that could explain the transition from mania to depression, but only one could explain all aspects of this unique mental illness. As described in Chapters 9 and 10, uncontrolled flooding of K^+ ions outside serotonin neurons can explain mania onset, a transition to temporary depression, euthymia, and a tendency for permanent cycling between mania and depression. There are many possible causes of K^+ flooding, including increased levels of Ca^{++} in cytosol and impaired astrocyte clearance of K^+ ions. As described in Chapter 10, the switch to depression begins when brain function becomes dominated by a sharp decline in serotonin activity. This mechanism was reported in May 2018 at the American Psychiatric Association Annual Meeting in New York City.[268]

Recovery from Depression: The major decline in serotonin activity at depression onset involves sharply reduced K^+ outflow while surviving clearance mechanisms continue to operate, resulting in slow and gradual removal of excess K^+ ions outside serotonin neurons. The return to mania is delayed by activity-inhibiting adaptations that developed during the previous mania phase that can be slow to fade away. The depression phase likely transitions to euthymia as extracellular K^+ concentrations approach 3 mM/L.

Euthymia and the Return of Mania: The discovery that serotonin is the likely switching neurotransmitter suggests that euthymia may be the initial phase of bipolar disorder and not the final phase before the return of mania. These periods of relative wellness are a distinctive feature of the illness, and the cause and mechanisms have been debated for decades. Serotonin has a powerful inhibitory effect on several major transmitters. Bipolar disorder onset begins when cumulative damage to the collaborating team of ion channels alters behavior of numerous neurotransmitter systems. As described in Chapter 10, serotonin neurons apparently experience the most severe damage and develop non-stop $(K^+)_o$ flooding and shrinking resting potentials that cause initial neuronal hyperactivity followed by a major decline in activity. Initial hyperactivity of inhibitory serotonin neurons puts the brakes on dopamine, norepinephrine, and other major transmitters that may create a temporary euthymia-like condition that delays onset of mania. Severe mania develops as serotonin activity transitions to hypoactivity during progressive neuronal flooding. In the absence of successful treatment, mania tends to increase in severity as serotonin activity declines.

An Explanation for Permanent Mania/Depression Cycling: In the absence of successful treatment, the brain will tend to return to mania (and not normality) because the genetic and acquired ion channel impairments present at bipolar disorder onset have not been resolved. Also, continuing damage to DNA and brain cells after onset will progressively weaken regulation of serotonin neurons and strengthen the tendency for mania/depression switching.

The Complexity of Bipolar Disorder

Clinicians and researchers often complain about bipolar disorder's heterogeneity. Psychiatrists are challenged by vast differences in symptoms exhibited by their patients and the need to devise individualized treatment approaches. Researchers are not only confronted by bipolar 1, bipolar 2, and cyclothymia phenotypes, but also significant differences in neuronal behavior, connectivity, and biochemistry within each group. Heterogeneity is an intrinsic feature of bipolar disorder since the illness involves a multitude of different damaged ion channel combinations that may confer very different symptoms. We have more than 400 ion channels coded by our genes, and each has numerous potential SNP mutations that may or may not be present. This explains why the first 30 years of genetic research failed to identify a single gene that predisposed to bipolar disorder and why medications and other treatments frequently require trial-and-error. Except for identical twins, it is likely that a psychiatrist will never have two bipolar disorder patients with the exact same disorder.

Development of a New Bipolar Disorder Theory

Over the past 1,000 years, leading scientists have advocated simple solutions to complex phenomena. In the 14th century, a Franciscan friar and logician published a principle known as Occam's razor that favors selection of theories with the fewest assumptions.[269,270] This has influenced Bacon, Boyle, Einstein, Newton, and others who compressed extreme complexity onto simplifying concepts such as $PV=nRT$, $E=mc^2$, and $F=ma$.[271,272,273] While at Princeton University, Einstein proposed a modified razor that has been paraphrased as "make things as simple as possible, but no simpler." I believe this approach applies to the extraordinary complexity of bipolar disorder. While recent years have brought several thoughtful and impressive bipolar theories, it was exciting to identify the likely cause and primary mechanisms of the illness, especially since they lead to a simplified explanation of bipolar disorder with minimal assumptions.

In the history of science, progress has often been advanced by theories that attempt to explain poorly understood phenomena. In this spirit, I propose a new theory of bipolar disorder[274] that is based on the findings of this investigation.

A Comprehensive Theory of Bipolar Disorder
by William J. Walsh, PhD

Genetic Predisposition. Increased risk for bipolar disorder is caused by two coincident factors: Genetic weakness in the team of 400+ collaborating ion channel genes, and genetic tendency for accelerated DNA damage. These impairments usually are not sufficient to produce the illness during childhood or adolescence.

Bipolar Disorder Onset. Several years of continuing damage to ion channels and other brain areas eventually impairs regulation of several neurotransmitters, resulting in generalized neuronal hyperactivity. Serotonin neurons experience the greatest damage and develop progressive $(K^+)_o$ flooding due to incomplete $(K^+)_o$ clearance after action potentials. This causes shrinking K^+ gradients and rest potentials that initially increase serotonin activity, followed by a gradual transition to severe hypoactivity as $(K^+)_o$ levels become extreme.

Mania Onset. Mania onset may be delayed by initial hyperactivity of inhibitory serotonin neurons that temporarily limit activity of norepinephrine, dopamine, and other transmitters. This may create an euthymia-like period (absence of mania or depression) that may last for weeks or months until serotonin neurons transition to hypoactivity. Mania begins as norepinephrine, dopamine, and other excitatory transmitters develop abnormal hyperactivity as serotonin inhibition fades away. In the absence of effective treatment, some patients may experience severe mania symptoms including psychosis.

The Switch to Depression. Declining serotonin activity eventually dominates brain function and triggers the onset of depression that may be severe and continue for more than a year. Recovery of serotonin function occurs automatically due to reduced K^+ outflow and surviving clearance mechanisms that gradually eliminate extracellular $(K^+)_o$ flood levels.

The Return of Mania. As depression slowly fades away, the return to mania is delayed by activity-inhibiting adaptations that developed during the previous mania phase. Eventually serotonin neurons return to hyperactivity (and not normality) because the damage to ion channel genes at bipolar onset is permanent. A relatively quiescent euthymia phase returns as elevated serotonin activity again temporarily inhibits activity of other transmitters. Mania returns as norepinephrine, dopamine, and other excitatory transmitters develop abnormal hyperactivity as serotonin inhibition fades away.

Chronic Mania/Depression Cycling. In the absence of successful treatment, the tendency to switch between mania and depression may continue indefinitely and become more severe due to progressive DNA damage over time.

References

261. Lord, C. J., & Ashworth, A. (2012). The DNA damage response and cancer therapy. *Nature, 481*(7381), 287–294.
262. O'Connor, M. J. (2015). Targeting the DNA damage response in cancer. *Molecular cell, 60*(4), 547–560.
263. Lahtz, C., & Pfeifer, G. P. (2011). Epigenetic changes of DNA repair genes in cancer. *Journal of molecular cell biology, 3*(1), 51–58.
264. Maliszewska-Olejniczak, K., & Bednarczyk, P. (2024). Novel insights into the role of ion channels in cellular DNA damage response. *Mutation Research-Reviews in Mutation Research, 793*, 108488.
265. Chen, J., Potlapalli, R., Quan, H., Chen, L., Xie, Y., Pouriyeh, S., ... & Xie, Y. (2024). Exploring DNA damage and repair mechanisms: A review with computational insights. *BioTech, 13*(1), 3.
266. Panagopoulos, D. J., Karabarbounis, A., Yakymenko, I., & Chrousos, G. P. (2021). Human-made electromagnetic fields: Ion forced-oscillation and voltage-gated ion channel dysfunction, oxidative stress and DNA damage. *International Journal of Oncology, 59*(5), 1–16.
267. Anderson, K. J., Cormier, R. T., & Scott, P. M. (2019). Role of ion channels in gastrointestinal cancer. *World Journal of Gastroenterology, 25*(38), 5732.
268. Walsh, W. J. and de Vito R. A. *"A neuroscience theory of bipolar disorder."* Abstract P7–109, 2018 Annual APA Annual Meeting, New York.

269. Sober, E. (2015). *Ockham's razors: a user's manual.* Cambridge University Press.
270. Duignan, B. (2023). Occam's Razor. In *Encyclopedia Britannica.* Encyclopedia Britannica.
271. Herivel, J. (1965). *The Background to Newton's Principia: A Study of Newton's Dynamical Researches in the Years 1664–84.* Clarendon Press
272. Thorburn, W. M. (1915). Occam's razor. *Mind 24,* 287–288.
273. Einstein, A., & Calaprice, A. (2011). *The ultimate quotable Einstein.* Princeton University Press.
274. Walsh, W. J. *Bipolar Disorder: A Channelopathy Disorder [abstract].* 2024 Society for Neuroscience Annual Conference, Chicago, IL.

CHAPTER 12

Discussion

The bipolar theory described in Chapter 11 is composed of several elements with differing degrees of certainty. The highest degree of confidence belongs to the discovery that bipolar disorder's genetic predisposition is dominated by germline mutations in ion channel genes. Continuing progress in GWAS and other genomic studies are expected to confirm this result that was based on the exclusion analysis of early bipolar disorder genetic variants. This finding was not a great surprise since K^+, Na^+, Ca^{++}, and Cl^- ions have central roles in neuron firing and neurotransmissions, and many researchers previously suggested that bipolar disorder may be a channelopathy. However, the discovery that a genetic tendency for accelerated DNA damage is essential to the development of bipolar disorder was completely unexpected. It is becoming clear that misbehaving ion channels significantly impair DNA damage repair and that abnormally high rates of DNA damage are intrinsic to bipolar disorder and other channelopathies. The median age of bipolar disorder onset is 25 years, indicating that more than two decades of accelerated damage are typically required for the illness to develop.

An important breakthrough was learning that progressive flooding by extracellular K^+ ions could explain (a) onset of mania, (b) the transition to depression, and (c) a tendency for chronic cycling between mania and depression. Progressive K^+ flooding at a neurotransmitter system prominent in clinical depression would lead to continuously declining neuronal activity that could trigger a switch to bipolar disorder's depression phase. My interest in this model increased upon realizing that reduced K^+ outflow from neurons and surviving clearance mechanisms would automatically tend to eliminate K^+ flooding, explaining the end of bipolar disorder's depression phase and the return of mania. This led to the switching model and new bipolar disorder theory presented in Chapter 11. While K^+ flooding represents a valid explanation for mania/depression switching, there may be other mechanisms that could produce a similar effect. Although not 100% proven, the comparative analysis of major neurotransmitters in Chapter 10 indicated serotonin was the neurotransmitter responsible for mania/depression transitions. This was a surprise since prior research suggested that dopamine and norepinephrine were more closely associated with bipolar disorder. Future advances in brain science will provide additional clarity and certainty regarding the unique mechanisms of bipolar disorder.

Bipolar Disorder Phenotypes

It appears bipolar disorder can develop in virtually anyone born with major mutations in ion channel genes and a propensity for accelerated DNA damage. This democratic illness has been observed in all humanity whether rich or poor, educated or illiterate, outgoing or antisocial, liberal or conservative, and criminal or law-abiding. This mental illness may be a singular "additive" disorder that takes different forms depending on a person's biochemical individuality and mental tendencies. For example, the relative risk for bipolar 1 or bipolar 2 may be associated with unrelated tendencies for anxiety or depression. My clinical studies of 30,000+ patients indicated that hypermethylation typically involves norepinephrine hyperactivity and anxiety, while hypomethylation is associated with low serotonin activity and clinical depression. It is very likely that various concomitant anxiety or depression conditions impact the risk for bipolar 1 and bipolar 2 phenotypes. In the above example, hypermethylation may predispose to mania and a higher risk for bipolar 1, while hypomethylation may be associated with bipolar 2 and heightened depression. However, DNA's methyl content is only one of several biochemical or genetic factors that impact mania or depression.[275] For example, specific combinations of ion channel variants may confer different depression or anxiety tendencies. In summary, factors unrelated to bipolar disorder may impact the risk for bipolar 1, bipolar 2, and other forms of this "additive" illness.

Bipolar Disorder – A Progressive Illness

While there is disagreement about many aspects of bipolar disorder, there is consensus that the illness generally becomes more severe with advancing age.[276] Research studies consistently show reduced treatment effectiveness in the years following onset of the disorder.[277] In-house outcome studies for hundreds of our bipolar patients showed greatest improvements prior to age 30 but only modest progress after age 50. Treatments that are effective during early years of the illness often produce little or no benefit later in life. For years, researchers have attempted to identify the cause of this phenomenon. A popular but controversial kindling hypothesis has been debated for decades. The term kindling was coined in the 1960s when epilepsy researchers learned that electrically induced seizures in animals made them far more prone to new seizures.[278,279] Some have likened this to burning a few twigs that could eventually start a major fire (kindling). This concept led to a kindling theory of bipolar disorder[280] that attempted to explain onset after years of relative wellness and progressive severity with advancing age. Kindling advocates believed that bipolar's mania and depression episodes can incrementally and permanently damage the brain and progressively worsen the illness. However, several scientists have proposed more modern explanations for increasing severity of bipolar disorder with age. For example, Berk and colleagues presented an interesting staging model that describes gradual worsening of bipolar disorder after onset.[281] In another example, Robert Post updated his original kindling theory, suggesting physical and emotional stresses may alter epigenetic marks on DNA, histones, and microRNA that exacerbate the illness.[282]

While theories attempting to explain bipolar's gradual increasing severity have become more sophisticated and plausible, it appears that bipolar's genetic weakness in protecting DNA integrity is the primary cause of worsening trajectory of the illness. The heightened assault on DNA continues after bipolar onset, causing additional damage to the ion channel team. The net result is greater complexity and severity of the illness as the patient ages. Relentless, increasing DNA damage is an intrinsic feature of bipolar disorder, and this is the most compelling explanation for the progressive nature of the illness.

Treatment Opportunities and Challenges

Despite clinical advances over the past century, virtually all psychiatrists and researchers agree there is a critical need for improved bipolar disorder therapies. This investigation has identified approaches that may immediately benefit bipolar disorder patients, guide development of future clinical improvements, and lead to effective prevention. In addition, exciting new gene editing,[283] histone modification,[131] miRNA,[140] mRNA,[284] ubiquitination,[285] and other advanced technologies have the potential to revolutionize treatment of the illness.

The Promise of Antioxidant Therapies: The brain is highly vulnerable to oxidative stress due to its high oxygen requirement, modest antioxidant defenses, and high lipid content. Although the brain is only 2% of the body's weight, it consumes 20% of the body's oxygen. There is strong evidence that elevated oxidative stress and inflammation are typical features of bipolar disorder and contribute to severity of symptoms.[286,287,288] Several bipolar disorder studies have reported significant benefits from the antioxidant N-acetylcysteine.[289,290] Antioxidant therapies may provide immediate partial benefits by (a) reducing brain inflammation and oxidative overload and (b) slowing future DNA damage.[291] Commercially available chemical analysis markers can identify excessive rates of DNA damage. Guanine has the highest charge of the four DNA nucleotides, causing greater vulnerability to ROS free radicals. Fortunately, oxidized (damaged) guanine compounds are at measurable levels in blood and urine. For example, laboratory testing for 8-oxo-dG (8-Oxo-2'-deoxyguanosine) is a direct marker for excessive DNA damage rates.[292] Other laboratory markers for DNA damage and oxidative overload include OGG1 (8-oxo-guanine glycosylase),[293] nitrotyrosine,[294] glutathione peroxidase, metallothionein, and a Cu/Zn imbalance in blood. In summary, there are several valid blood and urine laboratory assays that can identify abnormal DNA damage rates that may be effectively treated using existing and advanced antioxidant therapies.

Oxidative stress is an imbalance between the production of free radicals and the body's ability to counteract or detoxify their harmful effects. A free radical has been described as a thief that damages cells, proteins, or DNA by stealing an electron. The 63 known human antioxidant genes are classified into three groupings: dismutases, peroxidases, and thiol redox proteins.[184,295] While cosmic radiation and environmental insults contribute to oxidative stress, the two greatest sources of DNA damage in the brain typically are (a) superoxide, which is a byproduct of normal mitochondria and immunity processes,[296] and (b) the Fenton reaction[297,298] between H_2O_2 and Fe^{++}. While superoxide can damage DNA, its greatest harm results from hydroxyl and ONOO- (peroxynitrite) radicals formed by reactions of superoxide with other chemicals. The Fenton reaction is a separate source of dangerous hydroxyl radicals that assault DNA, neurons, and glial cells. In healthy people, H_2O_2 is maintained at acceptable levels by catalase, glutathione peroxidase, and other genetically expressed antioxidants. However, there is clear evidence of abnormally elevated H_2O_2 levels in bipolar disorder that contribute to oxidative stress, inflammation, and accelerated DNA damage. The good news is that presently available antioxidant supplements can effectively treat H_2O_2 overloads and minimize the Fenton reaction's contribution to DNA damage. However, coping with superoxide and its reaction byprod-ucts is far more complex and challenging because these radicals are relatively impervious to catalase, glutathione, zinc, Vitamin C, and other common antioxidants.

Healthy brains are protected by three SOD genes that express enzymes that regulate superoxide levels.[299] These apoenzymes quickly absorb Cu^{++} or Mn^{+++} ions that may donate an electron to convert superoxide to relatively innocuous H_2O_2. I think of dismutase as a "one-two punch" that converts superoxide to H_2O_2 that is more easily normalized by common antioxidants. Cu/Zn SOD1 is primarily expressed in neuronal cytosol, Mn SOD2 in mitochondria, and Cu/Zn SOD3 outside neuron membranes, providing individualized protection at key neuronal sites.[300] However, published studies report excessive superoxide, OH-, and ONOO- levels in bipolar disorder patients, sug-gesting a pronounced weakness in SOD protection.[301,302,303] Oral Cu/Zn SOD1 and Cu/Zn SOD3 supplements are commercially available, but their effectiveness has been very limited by inefficient absorption and brief half-lives in the bloodstream. In addition, Mn SOD2 supple-ments have not been approved for human consumption at this writ-ing. Improved methods for increasing brain levels of Cu/Zn SOD1, Mn SOD2, and Cu/Zn SOD3 would greatly benefit bipolar disorder patients and are under active development.

While effective regulation of superoxide and related radicals may require several years of research, there are several presently-avail-able approaches that may minimize their harmful effects. As men-tioned previously, published studies have reported efficacy of NAC supplements in bipolar patients. Although NAC has little direct impact on superoxide, it increases levels of Mn SOD2 and supports effective-ness of the other SODs.[304] Abnormal Cu and Zn blood levels impair dismutase capability of SOD1 and SOD3,[305,306,307] and about 80% of our 1,500+ clinical bipolar disorder patients exhibited significant Cu or Zn imbalances. Many of these patients and their doctors reported some degree of improvement simply by normalizing Zn and Cu levels in blood. Metallothionein (MT) proteins have been shown to effectively deactivate superoxide, hydroxy ions, H_2O_2, and other forms of ROS.[308,309] Four metallothionein genes (*MT1, MT2, MT3, MT4*) express short thiol redox proteins that exhibit remarkable antioxidant properties. For example, metallothionein proteins are 300 times more effective than glutathione in scavenging H_2O_2.[310] Metallothionein has primary responsibility for regulation of Cu and Zn in the body, and a patented MT-promotion supplement has been used since year 2000 aimed at epigenetic normalization of Cu levels.[36,311,312]

In summary, robust antioxidant therapy that might include NAC, normalization of copper and zinc blood levels, and metallothionein enhancement may benefit most bipolar disorder patients. These presently available antioxidant approaches could result in immediate improvements by reducing oxidative stress and inflammation in the brain, along with minimizing DNA damage rates. Future development of superior antioxidant therapies may enable an end to bipolar's progressive severity with age. Bipolar patients could be tested periodically for oxidative overload and excessive DNA damage rates and treated appropriately. Finally, high-risk children with a family history of bipolar disorder may benefit from early infant screening for elevated oxidative stress and accelerated DNA damage.[313] Early antioxidant therapy would likely prevent many children from developing this devastating mental illness.

Pharmaceutical Approaches: The new bipolar disorder model involves potassium ion flooding outside serotonin neurons that results in mania onset, a temporary transition to depression, euthymia, and the return of mania. Flooding could result from either an increased K^+ outflow or impaired clearance after action potentials. For example, increased Ca^{++} levels in cytosol would increase K^+ ion outflow through calcium-gated potassium channels, and impaired neuronal and glial clearance mechanisms could weaken clearance of K^+ ions. If this model is correct, a direct and highly promising therapy might involve the development of drug medications designed to enhance stability of serotonin activity. Several neuronal and glial mechanisms promote clearance of extracellular potassium ions and may be attractive targets for drug therapy. Medications that limit Ca^{++} cytosol levels or K^+ outflow may be effective. In addition, several psychiatric medications have antioxidant properties, suggesting that pharmaceutical companies could develop bipolar drugs designed to include robust antioxidant protection.[314] In summary, the new understanding of genetic predispositions and mechanisms of the illness may provide a guide for developing more effective drugs for treatment of bipolar disorder.

Ion Channel Therapies: Opportunities to directly combat genetic weaknesses in the ion channel team are very limited at present. CRISPR and other gene editing approaches[315] are highly promising for disorders caused by a single misbehaving gene or, perhaps, a few wayward genes, although certainly not the multitude of ion channel variants and variant combinations associated with bipolar disorder. Future progress in gene-editing techniques may eventually enable selective replacement of multiple misbehaving ion channel genes, but this may require decades of research. However, CRISPR and other gene-editing techniques are useful in basic research studies seeking better understanding of bipolar disorder and its unique mechanisms.

Alternative epigenetic therapies[316] to adjust expression rates of impaired ion channel genes might block unwanted mutated proteins or increase production rates of weakened genes but would fail to restore proper (canonical) amino acid sequences. Unfortunately, successful editing of a gene team with thousands of potential impaired gene combinations is a very daunting challenge. In summary, gene-editing and epigenetic therapies to directly fix a complex genetically weakened gene team are unattractive in the near-term.

While gene editing of multiple ion channel variants is extremely challenging, researchers are developing promising ubiquitination (UBI) and SUMOylation approaches that may minimize the impact of severely damaged ion channels.[317,318] UBI and SUMO treatments are being designed to (a) identify sites of major damage, (b) recruit appropriate repair proteins, and (c) optimize the decision process that leads to either apoptosis, senescence, cancer, or continuing function of a cell.[319] While most UBI and SUMO research is presently aimed at cancer, this technology could lead to improved bipolar disorder treatments.

DNA Repair Approaches: As described in Chapter 8, accelerated DNA damage to ion channel genes may be a prerequisite for development of bipolar disorder and a major cause of progressive severity. All human cells are exposed to cosmic radiation, environmental sources of ROS, unwanted chemical adducts that attach to DNA, and endogenous oxidative stress. Our cells are protected by DNA repair processes that can cope with typical damage levels. At this writing, there are more than 250 known DNA repair genes that attempt to reverse the somewhat shocking amount of daily DNA damage.[320] Therapies to directly improve effectiveness of mutated DNA repair genes are not yet available. Future gene-editing therapies may eventually be practical if a limited number of misbehaving genes are responsible for most repair inefficiencies. However, editing DNA repair genes may be extraordinarily difficult since there are a multitude of different repair-gene variant combinations in bipolar disorder. Recent studies have reported major DNA repair deficits in bipolar populations, especially base excision repair (BER) impairments.[321] At present, the relative damage caused by malfunctioning DNA repair genes or impaired antioxidant protection genes is unknown. In summary, effective gene-editing and epigenetic therapies to improve DNA repair capability are intrinsically very difficult and unpromising in the near term.

Concomitant Disorders: Bipolar disorder is a unique illness that may afflict nearly anyone born with severe ion channel mutations. This singular illness may take different forms depending on unrelated inborn and acquired brain disorders that also may be present. As described previously, patients challenged by major depressive disorder may be more prone to bipolar 2, whereas a coincident anxiety or panic tendency may confer higher risk for bipolar 1. In addition, there are metal metabolism, hormonal, methylation, and other biochemical imbalances that may contribute mental impairments not related to bipolar disorder. It seems clear that improved bipolar treatment efficacy may result from correction of these concomitant chemical imbalances that may interfere with mainstream bipolar treatments or exacerbate symptoms.

A Look at the Future

Advances in genomic science are unlocking key information hidden in our DNA strands that could lead to effective prevention of bipolar disorder within a few decades. As science progresses, the functional role of every gene and collaborative gene family will be determined. It is very likely that future DNA screens of young children will identify abnormal weaknesses in ion channel and DNA repair genes that indicate extreme risk for this disorder. More than 20 years of accelerated DNA damage typically are required for development of the illness, and this provides a large window of time to provide advanced antioxidants that may effectively prevent the disorder.

Development of antioxidant approaches capable of regulating superoxide, hydroxyl, and $ONOO^-$ free radicals may be available within 5–10 years. A major challenge may be enhancement of SOD1, SOD2, SOD3, and other dismutase enzymes to prevent excessive superoxide levels in the brain. Management of bipolar-prone persons may include occasional 8-oxo-dG or other laboratory tests to screen for excessive DNA damage rates. In addition, people at a high genetic risk for bipolar disorder should avoid environments and diets that increase oxidative stress. It seems clear that bipolar disorder research aimed at prevention should become a major priority throughout the world. It is very possible this devastating illness may gradually disappear from society in the near future.

Future DNA, RNA, and epigenetic screening of young children will routinely identify an increased risk for numerous physical and mental disorders, including cancer, heart disease, schizophrenia, bipolar disorder, autism, liver disease, immune disorders, and other late-onset maladies. This information will likely lead to targeted antioxidant therapies that may effectively prevent most of these illnesses. Relentless damage to our 25 trillion DNA strands begins the day we are born, and the medical world will soon learn that protecting DNA integrity must be a primary focus of healthcare. We are in the early stages of a revolution that could eliminate many major illnesses from society. In addition, advanced DNA protection will effectively delay the aging process, enabling healthy lifetimes well beyond 100 years. These future improvements in the human condition will result from the inevitable marriage between genetics, epigenetics, and neuroscience.

References

275. Li, S., & Tollefsbol, T. O. (2021). DNA methylation methods: Global DNA methylation and methylomic analyses. *Methods, 187,* 28–43.

276. Kraepelin, E. (1921). *Manic-depressive insanity and paranoia.* E. & S. Livingstone.

277. da Costa, S. C., Passos, I. C., Lowri, C., Soares, J. C., & Kapczinski, F. (2016). Refractory bipolar disorder and neuroprogression. *Progress in Neuro-Psychopharmacology and Biological Psychiatry, 70,* 103–110.

278. Coppolo, A., & Moshe, S. L. (2012). Epilepsy. In M.A. Aminoff, F. Boller & D.F. Swaab (Eds.), *Handbook of clinical neurology.* Elsevier.

279. Goddard, G. V. (1967). Development of epileptic seizures through brain stimulation at low intensity. *Nature, 214*(5092), 1020–1021.

280. Post, R. M. (2007). Kindling and sensitization as models for affective episode recurrence, cyclicity, and tolerance phenomena. *Neuroscience & Biobehavioral Reviews, 31*(6), 858–873.

281. Berk, M., Post, R., Ratheesh, A., Gliddon, E., Singh, A., Vieta, E., ... & Dodd, S. (2017). Staging in bipolar disorder: from theoretical framework to clinical utility. *World Psychiatry, 16*(3), 236–244.

282. Post, R. M. (2020). How to prevent the malignant progression of bipolar disorder. *Brazilian Journal of Psychiatry, 42*(5), 552–557.

283. WHO Expert Advisory Committee (2021). *Human genome editing: Recommendations.* World Health Organization, Geneva.

284. Rohner, E., Yang, R., Foo, K. S., Goedel, A., & Chien, K. R. (2022). Unlocking the promise of mRNA therapeutics. *Nature biotechnology, 40*(11), 1586–1600.

285. Weathington, N. M., & Mallampalli, R. K. (2014). Emerging therapies targeting the ubiquitin proteasome system in cancer. *The Journal of clinical investigation, 124*(1), 6–12.

286. Andreazza, A. C., Kauer-Sant'Anna, M., Frey, B. N., Bond, D. J., Kapczinski, F., Young, L. T., & Yatham, L. N. (2008). Oxidative stress markers in bipolar disorder: a meta-analysis. *Journal of affective disorders, 111*(2–3), 135–144.

287. Benedetti, F., Aggio, V., Pratesi, M. L., Greco, G., & Furlan, R. (2020). Neuroinflammation in bipolar depression. *Frontiers in psychiatry, 11,* 71.

288. Hassan, W., Noreen, H., Castro-Gomes, V., Mohammadzai, I., Batista Teixeira da Rocha, J., & Landeira-Fernandez, J. (2016).

Association of oxidative stress with psychiatric disorders. *Current pharmaceutical design, 22*(20), 2960–2974.

289. Berk, M., Malhi, G. S., Gray, L. J., & Dean, O. M. (2013). The promise of N-acetylcysteine in neuropsychiatry. *Trends in pharmacological sciences, 34*(3), 167–177.

290. Nery, F. G., Li, W., DelBello, M. P., & Welge, J. A. (2021). N-acetylcysteine as an adjunctive treatment for bipolar depression: A systematic review and meta-analysis of randomized controlled trials. *Bipolar disorders, 23*(7), 707–714.

291. Muneer, A. (2015). Bipolar disorder: role of inflammation and the development of disease biomarkers. *Psychiatry investigation, 13*(1), 18.

292. Hahm, J. Y., Park, J., Jang, E. S., & Chi, S. W. (2022). 8-Oxoguanine: from oxidative damage to epigenetic and epitranscriptional modification. *Experimental & molecular medicine, 54*(10), 1626–1642.

293. Ceylan, D., Yılmaz, S., Tuna, G., Kant, M., Er, A., Ildız, A., ... & Özerdem, A. (2020). Alterations in levels of 8-Oxo-2'-deoxyguanosine and 8-Oxoguanine DNA glycosylase 1 during a current episode and after remission in unipolar and bipolar depression. *Psychoneuroendocrinology, 114*, 104600.

294. Bandookwala, M., & Sengupta, P. (2020). 3-Nitrotyrosine: a versatile oxidative stress biomarker for major neurodegenerative diseases. *International Journal of Neuroscience, 130*(10), 1047–1062.

295. Gelain, D. P., Dalmolin, R. J., Belau, V. L., Moreira, J. C., Klamt, F., & Castro, M. A. (2009). A systematic review of human antioxidant genes. *Frontiers in Bioscience, 14*(12), 4457–4463.

296. Hayyan, M., Hashim, M. A., & AlNashef, I. M. (2016). Superoxide ion: generation and chemical implications. *Chemical reviews, 116*(5), 3029–3085.

297. Gutteridge, J. M., Maidt, L., & Poyer, L. (1990). Superoxide dismutase and Fenton chemistry. Reaction of ferric-EDTA complex and ferric-bipyridyl complex with hydrogen peroxide without the apparent formation of iron (II). *Biochemical Journal, 269*(1), 169–174.

298. Mao, G. D., Thomas, P. D., Lopaschuk, G. D., & Poznansky, M. J. (1993). Superoxide dismutase (SOD)-catalase conjugates. Role of hydrogen peroxide and the Fenton reaction in SOD toxicity. *Journal of Biological Chemistry, 268*(1), 416–420.

299. Younus, H. (2018). Therapeutic potentials of superoxide dismutase. *International journal of health sciences*, *12*(3), 88.

300. Miao, L., & Clair, D. K. S. (2009). Regulation of superoxide dismutase genes: implications in disease. *Free Radical Biology and Medicine*, *47*(4), 344–356.

301. Kucuker, M. U., Ozerdem, A., Ceylan, D., Cabello-Arreola, A., Ho, A. M., Joseph, B., ... & Veldic, M. (2022). The role of base excision repair in major depressive disorder and bipolar disorder. *Journal of Affective Disorders*, *306*, 288–300.

302. Lv, Q., Hu, Q., Zhang, W., Huang, X., Zhu, M., Geng, R., ... & Yi, Z. (2020). Disturbance of oxidative stress parameters in treatment-resistant bipolar disorder and their association with electroconvulsive therapy response. *International Journal of Neuropsychopharmacology*, *23*(4), 207–216.

303. Maes, M., Landucci Bonifacio, K., Morelli, N. R., Vargas, H. O., Barbosa, D. S., Carvalho, A. F., & Nunes, S. O. V. (2019). Major differences in neurooxidative and neuronitrosative stress pathways between major depressive disorder and types I and II bipolar disorder. *Molecular neurobiology*, *56*, 141–156.

304. Mao, G., Goswami, M., Kalen, A. L., Goswami, P. C., & Sarsour, E. H. (2016). N-acetyl-L-cysteine increases MnSOD activity and enhances the recruitment of quiescent human fibroblasts to the proliferation cycle during wound healing. *Molecular biology reports*, *43*, 31–39.

305. Dashti, S. I., Thomson, M., & Mameesh, M. S. (1995). Effects of copper deficiency and Cu complexes on superoxide dismutase in rats. *Nutrition (Burbank, Los Angeles County, Calif.)*, *11*(5 Suppl), 564–567.

306. Liu, T., Liu, Y., Zhang, F., & Gao, Y. (2023). Copper homeostasis dysregulation promoting cell damage and the association with liver diseases. *Chinese Medical Journal*, *136*(14), 1653–1662.

307. Airede, A. K. (1993). Copper, zinc and superoxide dismutase activities in premature infants: a review. *East African medical journal*, *70*(7), 441–444.

308. Hussain, S., Slikker Jr, W., & ALI, S. F. (1996). Role of metallothionein and other antioxidants in scavenging superoxide radicals and their possible role in neuroprotection. *Neurochemistry international*, *29*(2), 145–152.

309. Achard-Joris, M., Moreau, J. L., Lucas, M., Baudrimont, M., Mesmer-Dudons, N., Gonzalez, P., ... & Bourdineaud, J. P. (2007). Role of metallothioneins in superoxide radical generation during copper redox cycling: defining the fundamental function of metallothioneins. *Biochimie, 89*(12), 1474–1488.

310. Min, K. S., Nishida, K., Nakahara, Y., & Onosaka, S. (1999). Protective effect of metallothionein on DNA damage induced by hydrogen peroxide and ferric ion-nitrilotriacetic acid. *Metallothionein IV*, 529–534.

311. Walsh W. J. and Usman A. L. (2007). "Nutrient supplements and methods for treating autism and for preventing the onset of autism." US Patent No. 7,232,575.

312. Vašák, M. (2005). Advances in metallothionein structure and functions. *Journal of Trace Elements in Medicine and Biology, 19*(1), 13–17.

313. Zou, Y., Kennedy, K. G., Grigorian, A., Fiksenbaum, L., Freeman, N., Zai, C. C., ... & Goldstein, B. I. (2022). Antioxidative defense genes and brain structure in youth bipolar disorder. *International Journal of Neuropsychopharmacology, 25*(2), 89–98.

314. Park, S. W., Lee, C. H., Lee, J. G., Kim, L. W., Shin, B. S., Lee, B. J., & Kim, Y. H. (2011). Protective effects of atypical antipsychotic drugs against MPP+-induced oxidative stress in PC12 cells. *Neuroscience research, 69*(4), 283–290.

315. Gutiérrez-Rodríguez, A., Cruz-Fuentes, C. S., Genis-Mendoza, A. D., & Nicolini, H. (2023). CRISPR/Cas9 genome editing approaches for psychiatric research. *Brazilian Journal of Psychiatry, 45*(2), 137–145.

316. Pisanu, C., Katsila, T., Patrinos, G. P., & Squassina, A. (2018). Recent trends on the role of epigenomics, metabolomics and noncoding RNAs in rationalizing mood stabilizing treatment. *Pharmacogenomics, 19*(2), 129–143.

317. Rotin, D., & Staub, O. (2011). Role of the ubiquitin system in regulating ion transport. *Pflügers Archiv-European Journal of Physiology, 461*, 1–21.

318. Kanner, S. A., Shuja, Z., Choudhury, P., Jain, A., & Colecraft, H. M. (2020). Targeted deubiquitination rescues distinct trafficking-deficient ion channelopathies. *Nature methods, 17*(12), 1245–1253.

319. Chen, X., Zhang, Y., Wang, Q., Qin, Y., Yang, X., Xing, Z., ... & Qi, Y. (2021). The function of SUMOylation and its crucial roles in the

development of neurological diseases. *The FASEB Journal, 35*(4), e21510.

320. Coon, E. A., & Benarroch, E. E. (2018). DNA damage response: Selected review and neurologic implications. *Neurology, 90*(8), 367–376.

321. Ceylan, D., Tuna, G., Kirkali, G., Tunca, Z., Can, G., Arat, H. E., ... & Özerdem, A. (2018). Oxidatively-induced DNA damage and base excision repair in euthymic patients with bipolar disorder. *DNA repair, 65*, 64–72.

APPENDIX A

Neuron Resting Potentials

In 1889, a young man named Walther Nernst submitted his doctoral thesis to Leipzig University in Germany. This work included derivation of the now-famous Nernst equation that has become a fundamental law of electrochemistry.[A1] His brilliant career included the establishment of the science of physical chemistry and the third law of thermodynamics that brought him the 1921 Nobel Prize in Chemistry. He was the first prominent scientist to value the work of a young Albert Einstein, who left Switzerland and moved to Germany to be near Nernst and other leading scientists. The Nernst equation determines the voltage resulting from a difference in an ion's concentration across a cell's semi-permeable membrane.

$$\text{Voltage} = \frac{RT}{nF} \ln\left(\frac{(X)_o}{(X)_i}\right)$$

- Voltage is the membrane potential in volts (joules per coulomb)
- R is the ideal gas constant (8.31 joules per Kelvin • mole)
- T is the temperature in Kelvins
- F is Faraday's constant 96,485 coulombs per mole
- n is the valence of ion X
- X_o is the extracellular concentration of the ion (moles per cubic meter)
- X_i is the intracellular concentration of the ion (moles per cubic meter)

For a system involving only one ion type, the Nernst equation gives the electrical voltage resulting from that ion's concentration difference (or gradient) across a semi-permeable membrane. However, a neuron's bilayer membrane has leak channels for potassium, sodium, and chlorine ions, and the individual ions have very different permeabilities that impact voltage. Table 1 shows typical ion concentrations across a neuron's membrane at rest.

Table 1. Typical Ion Concentrations across a Neuron Membrane (millimoles per liter)

Inside Axon	Outside Axon	Nernst Voltage
$K^+ = 400$	$K^+ = 20$	- 77 mV
$Na^+ = 60$	$Na^+ = 436$	+ 50 mV
$Cl^- = 30$	$Cl^- = 590$	- 75 mV

The Nernst voltages in Table 1 represent the theoretical voltage for each ion, assuming no other permeable ions are present. The Goldman equation allows calculation of a neuron's overall resting voltage by including the effect of the different permeabilities.[A2] At rest, there are two major factors that contribute to a neuron's equilibrium voltage: (a) diffusional forces that cause ions to flow "downhill" toward lower concentrations of that ion, and (b) the relative ease with which a specific ion can pass the membrane (permeability). For a system involving a single ion, Nernst voltage represents an equilibrium condition in which there is no net flow across the membrane. Due to the multiple ions involved, brain neurons do not develop equilibrium rest voltages, but rather steady-state rest voltages.

$$V_m = \frac{RT}{F} ln \left[\frac{p_K (K^+)_o + p_{Na} (Na^+)_o + p_{Cl} (Cl^-)_i}{p_K (K^+)_i + p_{Na} (Na^+)_i + p_{Cl} (Cl^-)_o} \right]$$

- V_m is the membrane resting potential (voltage).
- R is the universal gas constant.
- T is the temperature in Kelvin.
- F is Faraday's constant 96,485 coulombs per mole
- P is the ion's permeability.

- [ion]$_o$ is the extracellular concentration of that ion (moles per cubic meter).
- [ion]$_i$ is the intracellular concentration of that ion (moles per cubic meter).

The K$^+$ leak channels in a neuronal membrane far outnumber Na$^+$ leak channels, causing Na$^+$ permeability to be negligible. In addition, the Nernst voltage for Cl$^-$ is very close to a neuron's rest voltage, so its impact on rest voltage is quite minor. As a result, potassium ions dominate rest voltages and the Nernst equation for K$^+$ closely approximates a neuron's resting voltage.

$$\text{Neuron Rest Potential} \cong \frac{RT}{F} \, ln \, \frac{(K^+)_o}{(K^+)_i}$$

The Nernst and Goldman equations illustrate the dominant role of potassium ion gradients and permeability on resting voltages. If localized potassium flooding outside neurons becomes significant, resting potentials in that brain area would move nearer to the threshold voltage, resulting in neuronal hyperactivity that might produce mania. Evaluation of abnormal potassium ion behavior was an early focus of this investigation.

References

A1.   Archer, M. D., (2011). *Genesis of the Nernst Equation."* In ACS Symposium Series, Vol.390. Chapter 8 (114–126).

A2.   Goldman, M. N., (1943). "Potential, impedance, and rectification in membranes." *Journal of General Physiology, 27*: 37–60.

APPENDIX B

DNA Repair

Types of DNA Damage: As described in Chapter 6, our trillions of unstable DNA molecules are severely damaged and repaired thousands of times every day. The discovery of DNA repair processes in the early 1970s is credited to Tomas Lindahl, a Swedish-born scientist.[B1] His early academic career was far from distinguished, including a failing grade in chemistry, possibly since he was also pursuing a career as a jazz musician. After successful research appointments in the USA at Princeton and Rockefeller University, he joined the Karolinska Institutet medical university in Stockholm, where he became fascinated with the intrinsic instability of DNA. With the knowledge that each DNA molecule is damaged several times each minute, he concluded that DNA repair mechanisms must exist. Otherwise, cells could not continue to function for months or years, and daughter cells from mitosis would be abnormal if they existed at all. Lindahl was the first to isolate DNA ligase and DNA glycosylase molecules that are central to base excision and other repair mechanisms.[B2] Lindahl, Sancar, and Modrich were awarded the Nobel Prize in 2015 for their pioneering research on DNA repair.[B3] Figure B-1 displays the major types of DNA damage and their repair mechanisms.

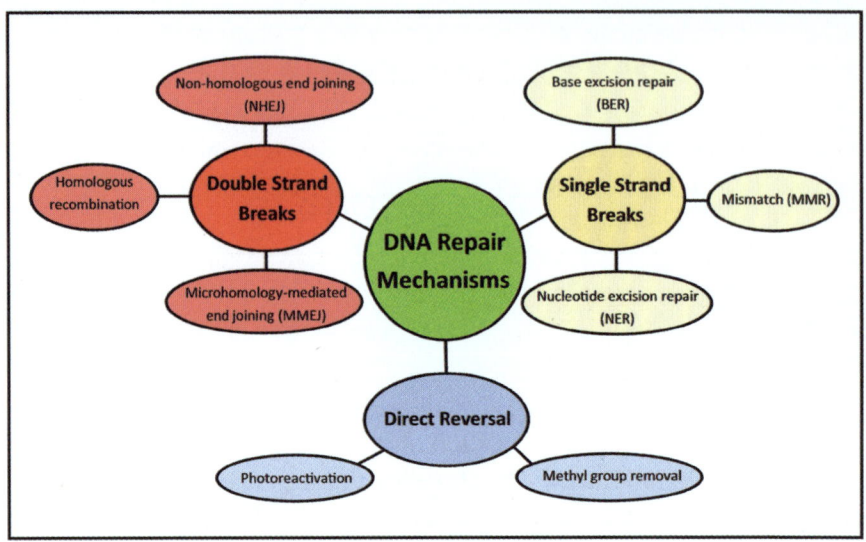

Figure B-1. Types of DNA Damage

Direct Reversal: This type of DNA repair can be achieved without removing the damaged base or breaking the DNA backbone. Each of the four DNA bases (adenine, cytosine, guanine, and thymine) may undergo an unwanted chemical reaction that can be quickly reversed. For example, methylation at guanine bases is directly reversed by the protein methyl guanine methyltransferase (MGMT).[B4] Methyl groups that attach to cytosine or adenine are efficiently removed by other methylase enzymes. Adjacent pyrimidine bases that covalently bond to each other due to UV radiation are quickly separated by photolyase enzymes. This type of DNA repair is especially effective against damage caused by UV light or alkylating agents.

Base Excision Repair (BER): In many cases, direct reversal fails to repair chemical reactions at a DNA base. While this defect usually doesn't alter the shape of the double helix, it can cause mutations or lead to breaks in DNA during replication. Guanine is especially vulnerable to oxidation by ROS because it has the highest charge of the four bases. Other chemical attacks on DNA include alkylated bases (3-methyladenine, 7-methylguanosine), deamination of adenine, and deamination of cytosine. These defects can be repaired efficiently by BER mechanisms.[B5,B6]

In the BER repair system, DNA glycosylases recognize the lesion and release the abnormal base by severing the N-glycosidic bond to form a single-strand break with a gap or nick in the damaged strand. The appropriate base is filled into the nick by RNA polymerase, guided by the corresponding base on the opposite strand that faces the nick. The nick is then sealed by DNA ligase to complete the repair process.

Nucleotide Excision Repair (NER): In the mid-1970s, Turkish-born scientist Aziz Sancar became fascinated by the recovery of bacteria which had been exposed to deadly amounts of ultraviolet (UV) radiation. His PhD thesis at the University of Dallas investigated photolyase enzymes that can repair DNA damage from UV-induced thymine-thymine bonding. Several years later at Yale, he discovered the basic NER mechanisms for the repair of DNA damaged by cosmic radiation.[B7,B8] He learned that UVrABC endonuclease enzymes can cut twice on human damaged DNA strands, removing 30 nucleotides that include the damaged segment. Since only one strand is damaged, RNA polymerase can perfectly replace the missing DNA segment, guided by the corresponding bases on the undamaged DNA strand.

DNA Mismatch Repair (MMR): Another type of damage involves DNA copying errors that result in a misplaced base that fails to correspond to the base in the opposing DNA strand. If not corrected, this mismatch could result in mutation, cell death, or cancer. Paul Modrich, a professor at Duke University, made many fundamental contributions to the understanding of DNA repair, with a focus on mismatch repair.[126,B9] Proofreading by RNA polymerase readily identifies mismatch after cell division, but an early problem was to determine which DNA strand was damaged. Modrich and colleagues solved the problem, recognizing that the daughter DNA had not yet been methylated. They later identified key mechanisms of mismatch correction, including the roles of MutH and other proteins, ATP activation, and the d(GATC) sequence that is capable of bidirectional excision. As in other types of single-strand DNA damage, insertion of proper replacement DNA bases is enabled by RNA polymerase. The original discoveries by Modrich's team came from studying DNA repair in bacteria. This work led to major advances in the understanding of human DNA repair.[B10]

Double-Strand Breaks: Most DNA damage involves single-strand defects that can be nicely repaired by BER, NER, or MMR mechanisms as summarized above. However, double-strand breaks occur frequently and must be quickly identified and repaired to ensure survival of the cell and cell line. Multiple double-strand breaks may appear on DNA strands after exposure to cosmic rays or other forms of ionizing radiation. Over many centuries, our cells have evolved two separate systems for repairing double-strand breaks: (a) homologous recombination (HR) and (b) non-homologous end joining (NHEJ).

Homologous Recombination (HR): This complex system for repairing double-strand breaks requires involvement of a sister DNA that serves as a template to guide repair.[B11] This can produce a perfect or near-perfect copy of the original undamaged DNA. The first step involves uncoiling of DNA from histones at the damage site to allow recruitment of special repair proteins. The stress caused by the DNA rupture activates JNK kinase that undergoes a phosphorylation reaction that essentially "identifies" or "signals" the DNA lesion and causes separation of the damaged DNA from its histone support structure. This provides access to SIRT6, PARP1, and ALC1/CHD1L proteins that begin to arrive within a second. These proteins collaborate to allow access to the DNA repair enzyme MRE11 that starts the repair process. In the first repair step, MRN complexes bind to DNA on either side of the break and, with other proteins, cut out the damaged segment. The remaining DNA strand is coated with a substance that enables interaction with an identical or very similar region of a nearby DNA. In a complex series of steps, the adjacent DNA strand is invaded with the appropriate segment cut out and inserted into the damaged DNA. The repair is completed by DNA ligase that seals the segment into the damaged DNA. The missing segment of the sister DNA is restored by RNA polymerase and sealed by DNA ligase. Homologous repair of double-strand breaks occurs less often than the end joining non-homologous alternative but does a more complete job of restoring DNA to its pre-damaged condition.

Non-Homologous End Joining (NHEJ): Most double-strand breaks are repaired by the NHEJ system that (a) identifies the lesion, (b) recruits proteins that remove the damaged segment, (c) trims the overhanging DNA at both ends, and (d) joins the ends back together without replacement of the damaged section.[B12] The first step involves attachment of MRN complexes at both of the broken ends that activate ATM proteins that form serine-threonine kinase dimers that provide robust phosphorylation to p53, histone 2a, and other proteins. Phosphorylated p53 acts as a transcription factor that can increase the concentration of RNA polymerase at promoter regions. These initial steps enable the formation of Ku heterodimer rings that surround both damaged ends. Artemis repair proteins attach to the Ku rings and enable precise cutting (removal) of DNA overhangs. The final step is the joining of the DNA ends by ligase IV (LIG4), xrcc4, and XLF proteins.

It's important to note that some DNA bases are lost after NHEJ repair. In most cases, the repaired DNA continues to function normally due to the tiny amount of DNA missing from the billions of bases comprising DNA. However, serious mutations may develop after (a) multiple NHEJ repairs or (b) if the lost DNA is an important part of a gene or promoter region.

Consequence of DNA Repair Failure: The ability of DNA repair processes to overcome the multitude of severe damage events is truly remarkable. However, the repairs are not perfect, and we gradually lose chromatin integrity over time, which is the primary cause of aging. As time passes, we can expect our cells to function less perfectly resulting in gray hair, skin wrinkles, and more serious impairments. Some cells may develop mutations that predispose to bipolar disorder or other mental illnesses. Complete failure of DNA repair has a devastating effect on a cell that may result in one of three following outcomes:

- Senescence: A state of dormancy in which the cell takes up space but ceases to function and cannot divide.[B13]
- Apoptosis: Cell suicide, usually followed by fragmentation and disappearance from the scene. [B14]
- Cancer: Uncontrollable division of abnormal cells that can spread throughout the body.[B15]

It is becoming clear that most cancers are caused by failed DNA repair. However, researchers have learned that cancer cells can be effectively killed by treatments that impair *their* DNA repair. Several promising DNA damage response cancer therapies are in FDA trials.[B16] It is fascinating that failed DNA repair can both cause cancer and be manipulated to kill cancer.

References

B1. Lindahl, T. (2013). My journey to DNA repair. *Genomics, proteomics & bioinformatics, 11*(1), 2–7.

B2. Huang, R., & Zhou, P. K. (2021). DNA damage repair: historical perspectives, mechanistic pathways and clinical translation for targeted cancer therapy. *Signal transduction and targeted therapy, 6*(1), 254.

B3. Cressey, D. (2015). DNA repair sleuths win chemistry Nobel. *Nature, 526*(7573), 307–308.

B4. Gutierrez, R., & O'Connor, T. R. (2021). DNA direct reversal repair and alkylating agent drug resistance. *Cancer Drug Resistance, 4*(2), 414.

B5. David, S. S., O'Shea, V. L., & Kundu, S. (2007). Base-excision repair of oxidative DNA damage. *Nature, 447*(7147), 941–950.

B6. Gohil, D., Sarker, A. H., & Roy, R. (2023). Base excision repair: mechanisms and impact in biology, disease, and medicine. *International journal of molecular sciences, 24*(18), 14186.

B7. Sancar, A., & Tang, M. S. (1993). Nucleotide excision repair. *Photochemistry and photobiology, 57*(5), 905–921.

B8. Marteijn, J. A., Lans, H., Vermeulen, W., & Hoeijmakers, J. H. (2014). Understanding nucleotide excision repair and its roles in cancer and ageing. *Nature reviews Molecular cell biology, 15*(7), 465–481.

B9. Kresge, N., Simoni, R. D., & Hill, R. L. (2007). Understanding DNA mismatch repair: the work of Paul L. Modrich. *Journal of Biological Chemistry, 282*(3), e2-e3.

B10. Li G. M. (2008). Mechanisms and functions of DNA mismatch repair. *Cell research, 18*(1), 85–98.

B11. Li, X., & Heyer, W. D. (2008). Homologous recombination in DNA repair and DNA damage tolerance. *Cell research, 18*(1), 99–113.

B12. Mao, Z., Bozzella, M., Seluanov, A., & Gorbunova, V. (2008). DNA repair by nonhomologous end joining and homologous recombination during cell cycle in human cells. *Cell cycle, 7*(18), 2902–2906.

B13. Shmulevich, R., & Krizhanovsky, V. (2021). Cell senescence, DNA damage, and metabolism. *Antioxidants & redox signaling, 34*(4), 324–334.

B14. Elmore, S. (2007). Apoptosis: a review of programmed cell death. *Toxicologic pathology, 35*(4), 495–516.

B15. Alhmoud, J. F., Woolley, J. F., Al Moustafa, A. E., & Mallei, M. I. (2021). DNA damage/repair management in cancers. *Advances in Medical Biochemistry, Genomics, Physiology, and Pathology*, 309–339.

B16. Li, Q., Qian, W., Zhang, Y., Hu, L., Chen, S., & Xia, Y. (2023). A new wave of innovations within the DNA damage response. *Signal transduction and targeted therapy, 8*(1), 338.

APPENDIX C

Exclusion Analysis of GWAS Variants

The exclusion analysis in Chapter 8 identified ion channel mutations as the primary cause of bipolar disorder. This discovery was based on GWAS consortium research that discovered 64 gene variants associated with elevated risk of the illness.[158,159] Table C-1 shows the specific SNP locations for each of these variants. After my investigation learned that bipolar disorder is a DNA damage disorder, it was essential to disregard DNA repair and antioxidant protection variants which obscure the search for true bipolar variants. The exclusion analysis compared each gene with respect to the following criteria:

- An important role in action potentials and neurotransmission.
- A strong association with cancer or other DNA-damage disorders.

Exclusion and inclusion decisions were quite straightforward for most variants, but more than 10% had significant associations with both criteria. For example, *CACNA1C* genes have a major effect on neuronal behavior, but also significantly increase risk for DNA damage.[C1,C2] In this example, *CACNA1C* was accepted because its powerful role in neurotransmission outweighs its lesser effect on DNA damage. This appendix also describes the function of the 63 genes and the intergenic variant in this analysis, based on the information available at this writing. However, these genes are still the subject of extensive research that may alter some of the exclusion/inclusion decisions in Chapter 8. In addition, many new bipolar variants will be discovered in future years. I expect advancing genetic science will confirm that impaired ion channels dominate genetic predisposition for bipolar disorder.

Table C1. Specific SNPs Identified in Connection with Bipolar Disorder

GENE	SNP Variants
ADCY2	rs28565152
ADD3	rs2273738
ADO	rs10761661
ANK3	rs10994415
BCL11B	rs2693698
C15orf53	rs35958438
C16orf72	rs28455634
CACNA1C	rs11062170
CACNB2	rs1998820
CD47	rs696366
CERS6	rs13417268
CUL4A	rs35306827
DOCK2	rs10866641
ERBB2	rs11870683
ERBB2	rs61554907
FADS2	rs174592
FKBP2	rs4672
FURIN	rs4702
GRIN2A	rs7199910
HDAC5	rs228768
HOMER1	rs6865469
HOMER2	rs62011709
Intergenic	rs2719164
ITIH1	rs2336147
KCNB1	rs237460
KDM3B	rs10043984
KIAA1109	rs112481526

GENE	SNP Variants
LINC01748	rs2126180
LMAN2L	rs4619651
MAD1L1	rs12668848
MDFIC2	rs115694474
MHC	rs13195402
miR124-1	rs62489493
MPP6	rs12672003
MRPS33	rs10255167
MSRA	rs3088186
NUF2	rs10737496
ODZ4	rs12289486
OSBPL2	rs13044225
PACS1	rs475805
PC	rs678397
PCGEM1	rs2011302
PLEC	rs6992333
PLXNA4	rs6946056
POU3F2	rs1487445
RP1-84O15.2 (lincRNA)	rs2953928
RPL13	rs12932628
RPS6KA2	rs10455979
RTN4RL1	rs4790841
SCN2A	rs17183814
SHANK2	rs12575685
SLC25A17	rs5758064
SP4	rs6954854
SRPK2	rs11764361
SSBP2	rs6887473
STARD9	rs4447398
STK4	rs67712855
SYNE1	rs4331993

GENE	SNP Variants
THSD7A	rs113779084
TRANK1	rs9834970
TUBBP5	rs62581014
WFDC12	rs6032110
ZCCHC7	rs10973201
ZNF592	rs748455

Most of the genes evaluated in the exclusion analysis have significant impacts on numerous brain mechanisms and functions. The following gene descriptions summarize known associations with (a) action potentials and neurotransmission or (b) DNA damage, but do not attempt to provide a comprehensive description of other roles in the brain.

ADCY2
ADCY2 codes for adenyl cyclase, a protein that catalyzes formation of cAMP, a second messenger essential for cell survival and neurotransmission pathways.[C3] It has many other important roles in synaptic plasticity and cell differentiation.

ADD3
Adducin 3 (ADD3) codes for γ-adducin, which functions as part of the assembly for the actin cytoskeleton. Dysregulation has been associated with increased tumor growth in glioblastoma multiforme.[C4] In addition, ADD3 alternative splicing is linked with lung cancer.

ADO
Cysteamine dioxygenase (ADO) preserves the homeostasis of oxygen and regulates thiol metabolism.[C5] It is found in the mitochondria, with predominant expression occurring in brain and muscle tissue.[C6] ADO's use of proline pairs enable it to be flexible in handling different sizes of substrates,[C5] and thus is critically important for regulation of oxidative stress.[C6] ADO has also been found to have a tumorigenic role in glioma.[C7]

ANK3
This was the first bipolar gene variant identified in high-population genetic studies and is regarded as a relatively strong contributor to

bipolar disorder risk compared to other small-effect variants. *ANK3* encodes an adaptor protein (ankyrin-G) that regulates the positioning of voltage-gated ion channels including placement of high concentrations of voltage-gated Na⁺ channels at AIS and nodes of Ranvier.[161,C8,C9,C10]

BCL11B
This B cell leukemia 11b (*BCL11B*) gene codes for a zinc finger protein transcription factor that is essential for life.[C11] This gene's expression is related to T cell development and function, including NK cell differentiation.[C12] It plays a complex role in cancer, acting as both a tumor suppressor and a potential oncogene.

C15orf53
This gene encodes for proteins that reside solely in immunological cells with a lack of expression in the limbic system.[C13] In addition, *C15orf53* has also been shown to be correlated with symptom counts of alcoholism, along with its presence in GWAS studies showing it to be correlated with BD as well.[C14] This gene has also been associated with worse prognosis in breast cancer.[C15]

C16orf72
Cells with a deficiency of this gene appear to pose a severe threat to stability in the loss of telomere homeostasis.[C16] For this reason, some researchers have termed *C16orf72* as "Telomere Attrition and p53 Response 1."[C16] *C16orf72* is also known as *HAPSTR1* and has a functional role in the stress response of cells, such as in reaction to cancer and neurodegeneration.[C17]

CACNA1C
CACNA1C encodes the α1C subunit of the Cav1.2 voltage-dependent L-type calcium channel (LTCC), which works towards cell membrane depolarization and calcium flow.[C18] This gene expresses L-type voltage-gated calcium channels that open during depolarization causing an inrush of Ca⁺⁺ ions that trigger the spraying of neurotransmitters into a synapse. It also has a key role in activating K⁺ channels during repolarization (recovery from an action potential), along with numerous other important roles in neurotransmission.[162,C19]

CACNB2

This gene in humans codes for the auxiliary subunit β2 protein in calcium voltage-gated channels, which are primarily found in pyramidal neurons of the hippocampus.[C20] This L-type calcium channel is related to the excitability of neurons and their release of neurotransmitters through the regulation of calcium currents.[C20]

CD47

Cluster of differentiation 47 (CD47), previously known as integrin-associated protein (IAP), belongs to a family of genes and proteins responsible for work in the immune system.[C21,22] CD47 proteins bind to the surface of a cell as a way to mark which cells are to be consumed via phagocytosis, and overexpression of this gene is associated with numerous cancers, poorer prognosis, and shorter survival times.[C22]

CERS6

As a gene responsible for ceramide synthesis, it is known as a longevity associated gene (LASS).[C23,C24] CERS6 also plays a role in mitochondrial functions in relation to Ca^{++},[C25] affecting the cell's Ca^{++} gradient and impairing cell function and signaling ability.[C26,C27] It is associated with poor prognosis and increased metastasis of breast cancer.

CUL4A

CUL4A is a member of the cullin 4 gene subfamily which promotes ubiquitination of substrates.[C28] CUL4A specifically is important to DNA repair processes, and its expression rate will change depending on the phase of the cell cycle, with high expression during S phase.[C28] Overexpression is associated with tumor growth and metastasis in breast, lung, and colorectal cancers.

DOCK2

DOCK2 has a role in numerous important cellular processes from migration and proliferation to immune function and response to ROS.[C29] One of the ways in which DOCK2 does these things through a role in the DNA damage response.[C30] The DOCK2 gene is implicated in numerous cancers.

ERBB2

While literature is sparse on the individual SNPs associated with BD for this gene, *ERBB2* is well known as *HER2*, a proto-oncogene.[C31] *HER2* is primarily associated with breast cancer, and its overexpression can be used as a predictor of severity due to its heterodimer's important role in cell cycle regulation.[C32]

FADS2

FADS2 is a gene highly expressed in the brain.[C33] It plays an important role in LC-PUFA metabolism, and this has been shown to potentially impact cognitive function.[C34] *FADS* is closely associated with breast cancer occurrence and development.[C35]

FKBP2

FK506-binding protein 2 (FKBP2), an ER-resident proline isomerase, may be required for proper proinsulin folding.[C36] A deficiency in the gene or a misfolding of its protein may result in apoptosis of the cell through Ca^{++} communication in the cell.[C36] *FKBP2* is associated with kidney cancer.[C37]

FURIN

This gene codes for Furin, a serine protease, which cleaves substrates and amino acid motifs in order to activate important molecules such as hormones, growth factors, enzymes and more.[C38] Anomalous expression can lead to malignant tumor growth.[C38]

GRIN2A

This gene encodes the NR2A subunit of the NMDA receptor, which works to bind glutamate.[C39] Disruption of the subunit can lead to disruption of the flow of Ca^{++} and Mg^{++}, and this can lead to a number of neurodevelopmental disorders and epilepsy.[C39,C40]

HDAC5

Histone-deacetylase 5 (*HDAC5*) works through epigenetic mechanisms and is involved in memory consolidation.[C41] Part of *HDAC5*'s function relates to heterochromatin maintenance in S phase of the cell cycle, which can lead to autophagy and apoptosis of cancer cells.[C42]

HOMER1
This gene is from a family that deals with synaptic plasticity, specifically in cases of glutamate transmission.[C43] In order for *HOMER1* to transcribe its protein, it requires the neuron to be stimulated.[C44]

HOMER2
The Homer family of proteins work as scaffolding proteins to bind different receptors,[C45] and as such are crucial for the regulation of synaptic plasticity, specifically with glutamate signalling.[C46] *HOMER2* also has diagnostic importance in cancer, specifically HBV-HCC, through its relation to tumor differentiation grade.[C47]

Intergenic
Intergenic is a unique case, because it refers not to a gene, but the region between genes. These areas may help to regulate gene expression through binding sites for transcription factors and enhancers.[C48] The specifically noted variant rs2719164 associated with BD is found on chromosome 2, between the genes *SEC61GP1* and *DNAJC17P*. [C49,C50] These genes are related to tumorigenesis[C51] and transcription splicing[C52] processes respectively.

ITIH1
ITIH1 is from a family of genes that code for protease inhibitors, which are associated with the extracellular matrix.[C53,C54] *ITIH1* is also correlated with checkpoint genes in a variety of cancer types.[C53]

KCNB1
This gene codes for a voltage-gated K^+ channel heavily involved integrin K^+ channel complexes (IKCs). Mutations in *KCNB1* and thus problems in the IKCs can lead to dysregulation of cellular functions, as well as developmental abnormalities.[C55]

KDM3B
KDM3B is a gene that codes for a protein in a family of demethylases. This means the protein's main role is in affecting the epigenetics of the DNA around it. As a result, a dysregulation of *KDM3B*'s normal expression can lead to a variety of effects, including an increase or decrease in likelihood of tumors depending on the context in which the gene has been affected.[C56]

KIAA1109

KIAA1109 has exhibited a major impact on survival rates in mouse and fruit fly studies.[C57,C58] In addition, it is associated with regulation of specific cancers. Mutations in this gene region lead to a greater percentage of survival time for patients with endometrial cancer.[C59]

LINC01748

This gene codes for a long intergenic non-protein coding RNA molecule.[C60] It is from a family of transcripts that control gene expression at various transcriptional levels.[C60] LINC01748 is also associated with expression, tumor growth, and a lowered overall survival rate in non-small-cell lung cancer (NSCLC).[C61]

LMAN2L

LMAN2L proteins modulate glycoprotein interactions in the brain.[C62,C63] This leads to associations with various disorders including bipolar disorder, as well as correlations with intellectual disability.[C62]

MAD1L1

MAD1L1, or human MAD1 mitotic arrest deficient-like 1, is involved in the maintenance for spindle checkpoints during mitosis.[C64] Degradation of function can lead to instability in chromosomes during this important step.[C65] As such, it plays a role in tumor suppression and has been implicated in prostate and breast cancers.[C66]

MDFIC2

This gene domain primarily functions as an inhibitor to another region, the MyoD family.[C67] MDFIC2 can increase chemoresistance to certain cancer stem cells after interaction with β-catenin, a protein known to affect transcription regulation.[C68]

MHC

This gene coding region is known as the Major Histocompatibility Complex which codes for a variety of functional genes.[C69] Some of the proteins produced by this region have an inhibiting effect on natural killer cells and their role in the DNA damage response pathway.[C70] Altered MHC expression can allow cancer cells to evade immune surveillance and promote tumor growth.

miR124-1

This class of microRNA has been found to be specific to the brain and an important factor in neuronal synaptic plasticity,[C71,C72] and its activity is crucial in mature microglia developing functionally.[C73] miR124 has also been identified to have tumor suppressant functions in multiple cancer types.[C74]

MPP6

This gene codes for an RNA binding protein in the nucleus that is responsible for processing and trimming pre-mRNAs and tRNAs that were improperly coded.[C75,C76] MPP6 also is associated with poor outcomes in hepatocellular carcinoma, angiogenesis, and immune evasion in HCC.[C77]

MRPS33

This gene is from a family of genes responsible for coding human mitochondrial ribosomal proteins for the small subunit (MRPS).[C78] These proteins may play a role in shielding the ribosomal RNA from ROS in the mitochondria,[C78] as well as comprising a portion of mitoribosomal translation.[C79] At least one variant can cause epilepsy (neuronal hyperactivity).

MSRA

Methionine sulfoxide reductase (MSRA) repairs damage to proteins done by ROS.[C80] Lack or reduction of MSRA can lead to a host of issues, such as premature aging leading to a shortened lifespan and neurological deficits.[C80] MSRA has a role in ROS scavenging and has been associated with breast cancer.[C81]

NUF2

NUF2 has been implicated in decreasing survival rates in those with NSCLC (lung cancer) due to impaired regulation of cell proliferation and death.[C82] Mutations within this gene affect the checkpoint processes that cells undergo during mitosis, leading to dysregulated growth and worse outcomes in NSCLC.[C82] Overexpression of this gene has also been observed in breast and ovarian cancers.

ODZ4

This gene codes for a member of the teneurin family, a group of cell surface proteins involved in signaling as type II transmembrane receptors and neuronal pathfinders.[C83,C84] OZD4 also has a risk variant that affects how rewards are processed within the amygdala, and this is theorized to affect processing in people affected by bipolar disorder.[C85] Dysregulated ODZ4 genes are involved in neuroblastoma tumor development.[C86]

OSBPL2

Oxysterol binding protein like 2, also known as oxysterol binding protein-related protein 4, is part of a family of intracellular lipid receptors that binds sterols.[C87,C88] This molecule is important in regulating signaling for cell proliferation at the plasma membrane.[C88] This gene family has also been implicated in different liver cancers.[C89]

PACS1

This trans-Golgi-membrane traffic regulator is primarily active during brain development for an embryo, with its activity dropping off post-birth.[C90] PACS1, through its direction of various proteins, may have a role in promoting the migration and specification of cranial neural crest cells (CNCCs) during embryonic development.[C90] PACS1 plays a role in localizing neuron, vesicle, and glia membrane proteins, and this gene assists in ion channel regulation.

PC

This gene codes for pyruvate carboxylase, an enzyme that plays a role in glutamine synthesis.[C91] This is crucial for supply of the neurotransmitter glutamate.[C91,C92] PC also has an important role in cancer in lipid metabolism because of its protective function against oxidative stress.[C93]

PCGEM1

This gene expresses a long non-coding RNA that plays a notable role in tumor regulation[C94] by downregulating a microRNA tumor suppressor.[C95] Overexpression is observed in prostate, gastric, ovarian, and renal cancers.

PLEC

This gene encodes plectin, a protein family which functions as cyto-skeletal linkers.[C96] It is the only member of the plakin family to be expressed in astrocytes.[C97] A key function of plectin as a cytoskeletal protein is in vesicle trafficking, which is extremely important in neu-ronal signaling.[C97] PLEC has also been noted as a gene indicating susceptibility for testicular cancer.[C98]

PLXNA4

Plexin A4, or PLXNA4, seems to be correlated with expression of proteins that maintain the integrity of a cell's border and morphology.[C99] This has been proposed to have an impact in the mechanisms per-taining to axonal guidance in brain disorders.[C100] If PLXNA4 expres-sion is silenced, the proliferation of cancer cells is inhibited, though seemingly without relation to changes in the organization of the cyto-skeleton.[C101]

POU3F2

This gene is involved with transcription factors relating to neuronal cell differentiation.[C102] In mice, this is primarily displayed in the adult hippocampus.[C103] POU3F2 is highly linked to tumor progression in melanoma as well.[C104]

RP1-84O15.2 (lincRNA)

LincRNA, otherwise known as long intergenic noncoding RNA, is a component of the genome that may work to regulate expres-sion of nearby genes, though the lincRNA's function can vary wildly depending on tissue location and proximity to coding regions.[C105] This gene encodes RNA proteins, and its variants have been implicated in muscular dystrophy, bipolar disorder, schizophrenia, and ADHD. At this writing, the variant's specific role in bipolar disorder risk is unclear.[159,C106]

RPL13

This gene codes for the ribosomal protein eL13, which constitutes a portion of the 60S ribosomal subunit crucial to pre-ribosomal RNA processing.[C107] This affects protein synthesis, and can have an effect on the stability of p53, an important tumor suppressor.[C108]

RPS6KA2

This gene is involved in the MAPK signaling pathway that regulates cell growth, differentiation, and survival. Its functions include suppression of ovarian cancer cells by causing arrest in the G1 phase of the cell cycle.[C109]

RTN4RL1

This gene, known as Reticulon-4 Receptor-Like 1, codes for a member of the Nogo receptor family that restricts the growth of axons and excitatory synapses.[C110] RTN4 also plays a role in carcinogenesis, and lower RTN4 expression was found to be related to better survival outcomes in multiple cancer types.[C111]

SCN2A

This gene is responsible for encoding a sodium channel in neurons. Dysfunction in this channel can affect neuronal communication and lead to different disorders depending on if the issue was caused by a gain or loss of function mutation in the gene.[C112]

SHANK2

This gene codes for scaffolding proteins found on the dendrites of post-synaptic excitatory neurons involved in glutaminergic responses.[C113] SHANK2 has been linked with intellectual disability[C114] and other neuropsychiatric disorders such as bipolar disorder, due to the change of composition and thus function of specific receptors.[C115] SHANK2 also functions as a tumor suppressant by inhibiting growth of neuroblastoma cells.[C116]

SLC25A17

This gene (solute carrier family 25 member 17) is a member of the mitochondrial carrier superfamily SLC25, of which there are 53 different proteins.[C117] SLC25A17 is localized to the peroxisomal membrane and transports CoA, FAD, and NAD+, as well as PAP (adenosine 3',5'-diphosphate), FMN and AMP.[C118] Higher rates of SLC25A17 expression have been linked with the progression of triple-negative breast cancer through its modulation of ROS.[C119]

SP4

The SP4 protein is a transcription factor that controls the expression of other genes by binding to DNA in the form of a grouping of three zinc fingers.[C120] It is mostly expressed in neurons and linked to neuronal signaling and energy production.[C121] *SP4* also functions as a proto-oncogene which can contribute to cancer progression by interfering with microRNAs and other protective molecules.[C122]

SRPK2

This gene enables phosphorylation of pre-mRNA that may prevent issues while preparing and splicing the RNA.[C123] This phosphorylation is required to help suppress the formation of R-loops, which are accidental formations that lead to genomic instability during the transcription process.[C124] *SRPK2* is aberrantly expressed in human colorectal cancer.[C125]

SSBP2

This gene codes for sequence-specific ssDNA-binding protein 2 and is primarily known as a tumor suppressor gene.[C126] When this gene and its protein expression are disrupted and lost, there is a decrease in the ability to recover from cytotoxic stress, as well as changes in transcription associated with cancer growth.[C126,C127]

STARD9

STARD9, also known as *KIF16A*, is a part of the kinesin protein superfamily, and it codes for a 4,700 amino acid protein.[C128] Multiple studies have shown that depletion or improper formation of this protein can lead to problems with mitosis.[C128,C129] *STARD9*-depleted cancer cells display increased sensitivity to taxol and other chemotherapy drugs.[C130]

STK4

This gene, also known as *LKB1*, encodes a serine/threonine kinase which helps regulate cell growth, polarity, and energy metabolism.[C131] This kinase is associated with several cancers due to phosphorylation of *p53*, a tumor suppressor gene.[C132]

SYNE1

This large gene is known to encode multiple proteins, including CPG2, which is a protein specifically localized at postsynaptic sites of excitatory synapses.[C133] This protein assists regulation of glutamate receptors.[C133,C134] Mutations in SYNE1 have been associated with ovarian cancer.[C135]

THSD7A

This gene encodes an N-glycoprotein that assists growth of new brain vascular pathways from older blood vessels by cell migration and cytoskeletal reorganization.[C136] Overexpression of this gene has been associated with prostate cancer, while lack of the gene correlated with colorectal and renal carcinomas.[C137]

TRANK1

TRANK1 is highly associated with genes and processes that affect neurotransmission, such as the growth and placement of synaptic pathways.[C138] Although not implicated in cancers, TRANK1 is strongly associated with antioxidant capability and protection against DNA damage.[C139]

TUBBP5

This gene encodes a beta-tubulin protein, a key component of microtubules that are essential for cell structure and movement.[C140] The Tubb5 protein is associated with several neurodevelopmental disorders and been identified as a somatic expression quantitative trait locus (eQTL) in various cancers.[C141]

WFDC12

This gene encodes a protease inhibitor that tends to increase the half-life of expressed proteins and has a role in inflammation and immune functions.[C142] While an SNP-weakened WFDC12 variant could increase DNA damage, it appears to have a greater role in ion channel behavior and regulation of neuronal activity.[167]

ZCCHC7

ZCCHC7's function lies in RNA degradation.[C143] It works with other protein complexes to affect telomerase RNA, a protective factor that maintains the ends of chromosomes.[C144] ZCCHC7 has also been linked with lymphomas.[C145]

ZNF592

This zinc-finger gene codes a protein 1,267 amino acids long which contains an extremely common eukaryotic DNA-binding motif.[C146] It is expected to have an important role in transcriptional regulation and other processes that involve the interaction between DNA and proteins.[C146] There is evidence that *ZNF592* may have a major influence on ion channel activity in cerebellum and substantia nigra (primary site of dopamine neurons).

References

C1.   Gakenheimer-Smith, L., Meyers, L., Lundahl, D., Menon, S. C., Bunch, T. J., Sawyer, B. L., ... & Etheridge, S. P. (2021). Expanding the phenotype of CACNA1C mutation disorders. *Molecular Genetics & Genomic Medicine, 9*(6), e1673.

C2.   Napolitano, C., & Priori, S. G. (2024). CACNA1C-related disorders. *GeneReviews®[Internet]*.

C3.   Stelzer, G., Rosen, N., Plaschkes, I., Zimmerman, S., Twik, M., Fishilevich, S., ... & Lancet, D. (2016). The GeneCards suite: from gene data mining to disease genome sequence analyses. *Current protocols in bioinformatics, 54*(1), 1–30.

C4.   Tan, Y., Xu, F., Xu, L., & Cui, J. (2022). Long non-coding RNA LINC01748 exerts carcinogenic effects in non-small cell lung cancer cell lines by regulating the microRNA-520a-5p/HMGA1 axis. *International Journal of Molecular Medicine, 49*(2), 1–15.

C5.   Li, X., Zhang, L., Yi, Z., Zhou, J., Song, W., Zhao, P., ... & Ni, Q. (2022). NUF2 Is a Potential Immunological and Prognostic Marker for Non-Small-Cell Lung Cancer. *Journal of Immunology Research, 2022*(1), 1161931.

C6.   Alkhater, R. A., Wang, P., Ruggieri, A., Israelian, L., Walker, S., Scherer, S. W., ... & Minassian, B. A. (2019). Dominant LMAN2L mutation causes intellectual disability with remitting epilepsy. *Annals of Clinical and Translational Neurology, 6*(4), 807–811.

C7.   Levchenko, A., & Plotnikova, M. (2023). Genomic regulatory sequences in the pathogenesis of bipolar disorder. *Frontiers in Psychiatry, 14*, 1115924.

C8.   Sanders, S. J., Campbell, A. J., Cottrell, J. R., Moller, R. S., Wagner, F. F., Auldridge, A. L., ... & Bender, K. J. (2018). Progress in understanding and treating SCN2A-mediated disorders. *Trends in neurosciences, 41*(7), 442–456.

C9.   Holmes, R. S., Barron, K. A., & Krupenko, N. I. (2018). Ceramide synthase 6: Comparative analysis, phylogeny and evolution. *Biomolecules, 8*(4), 111.

C10.   Shi, Y., Zhou, C., Lu, H., Cui, X., Li, J., Jiang, S., ... & Zhang, R. (2020). Ceramide synthase 6 predicts poor prognosis and activates the AKT/mTOR/4EBP1 pathway in high-grade serous ovarian cancer. *American journal of translational research, 12*(9), 5924.

C11.   Novgorodov, S. A., Chudakova, D. A., Wheeler, B. W., Bielawski, J., Kindy, M. S., Obeid, L. M., & Gudz, T. I. (2011). Developmentally regulated ceramide synthase 6 increases mitochondrial Ca2+ loading capacity and promotes apoptosis. *Journal of Biological Chemistry, 286*(6), 4644–4658.

C12.   Brini, M. (2003). Ca2+ signalling in mitochondria: mechanism and role in physiology and pathology. *Cell Calcium, 34*(4–5), 399–405.

C13.   Glancy, B., & Balaban, R. S. (2012). Role of mitochondrial Ca2+ in the regulation of cellular energetics. *Biochemistry, 51*(14), 2959–2973.

C14.   Su, Y., Gu, X., Zheng, Q., Zhu, L., Lu, J., & Li, L. (2022). LncRNA PCGEM1 in human cancers: functions, mechanisms and promising clinical utility. *Frontiers in oncology, 12*, 847745.

C15.   Zhang, S., Li, Z., Zhang, L., & Xu, Z. (2018). MEF2-activated long non-coding RNA PCGEM1 promotes cell proliferation in hormone-refractory prostate cancer through downregulation of miR-148a. *Molecular Medicine Reports, 18*(1), 202–208.

C16.   Jaura, R., Yeh, S. Y., Montanera, K. N., Ialongo, A., Anwar, Z., Lu, Y., ... & Rhee, H. S. (2022). Extended intergenic DNA contributes to neuron-specific expression of neighboring genes in the mammalian nervous system. *Nature Communications, 13*(1), 2733.

C17.   O'Connell, K. S., Smeland, O. B., & Andreassen, O. A. (2022). Genetics of bipolar disorder. In *Psychiatric Genomics* (pp. 43–61). Academic Press.

C18.   Sollis, E., Mosaku, A., Abid, A., Buniello, A., Cerezo, M., Gil, L., ... & Harris, L. W. (2023). The NHGRI-EBI GWAS Catalog: knowledgebase and deposition resource. *Nucleic acids research, 51*(D1), D977-D985.

C19.   Jin, L., Chen, D., Hirachan, S., Bhandari, A., & Huang, Q. (2022). SEC61G regulates breast cancer cell proliferation and metastasis by affecting the Epithelial-Mesenchymal Transition. *Journal of Cancer, 13*(3), 831.

C20. Pascarella, A., Ferrandino, G., Credendino, S. C., Moccia, C., D'Angelo, F., Miranda, B., ... & Amendola, E. (2018). DNAJC17 is localized in nuclear speckles and interacts with splicing machinery components. *Scientific reports, 8*(1), 7794.

C21. Li, W., Cai, X., Li, H. J., Song, M., Zhang, C. Y., Yang, Y., ... & Chang, H. (2021). Independent replications and integrative analyses confirm TRANK1 as a susceptibility gene for bipolar disorder. *Neuropsychopharmacology, 46*(6), 1103–1112.

C22. Haridas, V., Ni, J., Meager, A., Su, J., Yu, G. L., Zhai, Y., ... & Aggarwal, B. B. (1998). Cutting edge: TRANK, a novel cytokine that activates NF-κB and c-Jun N-terminal kinase. *The Journal of Immunology, 161*(1), 1–6.

C23. Chang, Q. H., Mao, T., Tao, Y., Dong, T., Tang, X. X., Ge, G. H., & Xu, Z. J. (2021). Pan-cancer analysis identifies ITIH1 as a novel prognostic indicator for hepatocellular carcinoma. *Aging (Albany NY), 13*(8), 11096.

C24. Morcel, K., Watrin, T., Jaffre, F., Deschamps, S., Omilli, F., Pellerin, I., ... & Guerrier, D. (2013). Involvement of ITIH5, a candidate gene for congenital uterovaginal aplasia (Mayer-Rokitansky-Küster-Hauser syndrome), in female genital tract development. *Gene Expression, 15*(5–6), 207.

C25. Houser, J. S., Patel, M., Wright, K., Onopiuk, M., Tsiokas, L., & Humphrey, M. B. (2023). The inhibitor of MyoD Family A (I-MFA) regulates megakaryocyte lineage commitment and terminal differentiation. *Blood Cells, Molecules, and Diseases, 102*, 102760.

C26. Chen, C. J., Yang, C. J., Yang, S. F., Huang, M. S., & Liu, Y. P. (2020). The MyoD family inhibitor domain-containing protein enhances the chemoresistance of cancer stem cells in the epithelial state by increasing β-catenin activity. *Oncogene, 39*(11), 2377–2390.

C27. Oldenborg, P. A. (2013). CD47: a cell surface glycoprotein which regulates multiple functions of hematopoietic cells in health and disease. *International Scholarly Research Notices, 2013*(1), 614619.

C28. Lian, S., Xie, X., Lu, Y., & Jia, L. (2019). Checkpoint CD47 function on tumor metastasis and immune therapy. *OncoTargets and therapy*, 9105–9114.

C29. Liu, Y., & Lin, W. (2022). KIAA1109 is required for survival and for normal development and function of the neuromuscular junction in mice. *bioRxiv*, 2022–02.

C30. Gueneau, L., Fish, R. J., Shamseldin, H. E., Voisin, N., Mau-Them, F. T., Preiksaitiene, E., ... & Reymond, A. (2018). KIAA1109 variants are associated with a severe disorder of brain development and arthrogryposis. *The American Journal of Human Genetics*, *102*(1), 116–132.

C31. Qiao, Z., Jiang, Y., Wang, L., Wang, L., Jiang, J., & Zhang, J. (2019). Mutations in KIAA1109, CACNA1C, BSN, AKAP13, CELSR2, and HELZ2 are associated with the prognosis in endometrial cancer. *Frontiers in genetics*, *10*, 909.

C32. Devasani, K., & Yao, Y. (2022). Expression and functions of adenylyl cyclases in the CNS. *Fluids and Barriers of the CNS*, *19*(1), 23.

C33. Benedetti, F., Poletti, S., Locatelli, C., Mazza, E., Lorenzi, C., Vitali, A., ... & Colombo, C. (2018). A Homer 1 gene variant influences brain structure and function, lithium effects on white matter, and antidepressant response in bipolar disorder: a multimodal genetic imaging study. *Progress in Neuro-Psychopharmacology and Biological Psychiatry*, *81*, 88–95.

C34. Shiraishi-Yamaguchi, Y., & Furuichi, T. (2007). The Homer family proteins. *Genome biology*, *8*, 1–12.

C35. Li, J., Kurasawa, Y., Wang, Y., Clise-Dwyer, K., Klumpp, S. A., Liang, H., ... & Nagarajan, L. (2014). Requirement for ssbp2 in hematopoietic stem cell maintenance and stress response. *The Journal of Immunology*, *193*(9), 4654–4662.

C36. Liang, H., Samanta, S., & Nagarajan, L. (2005). SSBP2, a candidate tumor suppressor gene, induces growth arrest and differentiation of myeloid leukemia cells. *Oncogene*, *24*(16), 2625–2634.

C37. Yoo, J., Kim, G. W., Jeon, Y. H., Lee, S. W., & Kwon, S. H. (2024). Epigenetic roles of KDM3B and KDM3C in tumorigenesis and their therapeutic implications. *Cell Death & Disease*, *15*(6), 451.

C38. Ji, L., Xu, S., Luo, H., & Zeng, F. (2022). Insights from DOCK2 in cell function and pathophysiology. *Frontiers in molecular biosciences*, *9*, 997659.

C39. Wu, M., Li, L., Hamaker, M., Small, D., & Duffield, A. S. (2015). DOCK2 Regulates DNA Damage Response and Modulates the

Sensitivity to Chemotherapeutic Agents in FLT3/ITD Leukemic Cells. *Blood*, *126*(23), 3668.

C40.   Goldberg, A. C., & Rizzo, L. V. (2015). MHC structure and function–antigen presentation. Part 1. *Einstein (Sao Paulo)*, *13*, 153–156.

C41.   Gasser, S., & Raulet, D. H. (2006). The DNA damage response arouses the immune system. *Cancer research, 66*(8), 3959–3962.

C42.   Chen, C., Meng, Q., Xia, Y., Ding, C., Wang, L., Dai, R., ... & Liu, C. (2018). The transcription factor POU3F2 regulates a gene coexpression network in brain tissue from patients with psychiatric disorders. *Science translational medicine*, *10*(472), eaat8178.

C43.   Zhao, G., Wei, Z., & Guo, Y. (2020). MicroRNA-107 is a novel tumor suppressor targeting POU3F2 in melanoma. *Biological Research*, *53*, 1–10.

C44.   Hashizume, K., Yamanaka, M., & Ueda, S. (2018). POU3F2 participates in cognitive function and adult hippocampal neurogenesis via mammalian-characteristic amino acid repeats. *Genes, Brain and Behavior*, *17*(2), 118–125.

C45.   Rathje, M., Waxman, H., Benoit, M., Tammineni, P., Leu, C., Loebrich, S., & Nedivi, E. (2021). Genetic variants in the bipolar disorder risk locus SYNE1 that affect CPG2 expression and protein function. *Molecular psychiatry*, *26*(2), 508–523.

C46.   Cottrell, J. R., Borok, E., Horvath, T. L., & Nedivi, E. (2004). CPG2: a brain-and synapse-specific protein that regulates the endocytosis of glutamate receptors. *Neuron*, *44*(4), 677–690.

C47.   Harbin, L. M., Lin, N., Ueland, F. R., & Kolesar, J. M. (2023). SYNE1 mutation is associated with increased tumor mutation burden and immune cell infiltration in ovarian cancer. *International Journal of Molecular Sciences*, *24*(18), 14212.

C48.   Bignone, P. A., Lee, K. Y., Liu, Y., Emilion, G., Finch, J., Soosay, A. E. R., ... & Ganesan, T. S. (2007). RPS6KA2, a putative tumour suppressor gene at 6q27 in sporadic epithelial ovarian cancer. *Oncogene*, *26*(5), 683–700.

C49.   Guo, Y., Zhang, X., Yang, M., Miao, X., Shi, Y., Yao, J., ... & Lin, D. (2010). Functional evaluation of missense variations in the human MAD1L1 and MAD2L1 genes and their impact on susceptibility to lung cancer. *Journal of medical genetics*, *47*(9), 616–622.

C50.   Tsukasaki, K., Miller, C. W., Greenspun, E., Eshaghian, S., Kawabata, H., Fujimoto, T., ... & Koeffler, H. P. (2001).

Mutations in the mitotic check point gene, MAD1L1, in human cancers. *Oncogene, 20*(25), 3301–3305.

C51.   Tsukasaki, K., Miller, C. W., Greenspun, E., Eshaghian, S., Kawabata, H., Fujimoto, T., ... & Koeffler, H. P. (2001). Mutations in the mitotic check point gene, MAD1L1, in human cancers. *Oncogene, 20*(25), 3301–3305.

C52.   Kuo, M. W., Wang, C. H., Wu, H. C., Chang, S. J., & Chuang, Y. J. (2011). Soluble THSD7A is an N-glycoprotein that promotes endothelial cell migration and tube formation in angiogenesis. *PloS one, 6*(12), e29000.

C53.   Stahl, P. R., Hoxha, E., Wiech, T., Schröder, C., Simon, R., & Stahl, R. A. (2017). THSD7A expression in human cancer. *Genes, Chromosomes and Cancer, 56*(4), 314–327.

C54.   Hagen, G., Dennig, J., Preiß, A., Beato, M., & Suske, G. (1995). Functional Analyses of the Transcription Factor Sp4 Reveal Properties Distinct from Sp1 and Sp3 (*). *Journal of Biological Chemistry, 270*(42), 24989–24994.

C55.   Sheehan, K., Lee, J., Chong, J., Zavala, K., Sharma, M., Philipsen, S., ... & Schumacher, M. (2019). Transcription factor Sp4 is required for hyperalgesic state persistence. *PloS one, 14*(2), e0211349.

C56.   Safe, S. (2023). Specificity proteins (sp) and Cancer. *International Journal of Molecular Sciences, 24*(6), 5164.

C57.   Milligan, L., Decourty, L., Saveanu, C., Rappsilber, J., Ceulemans, H., Jacquier, A., & Tollervey, D. (2008). A yeast exosome cofactor, Mpp6, functions in RNA surveillance and in the degradation of noncoding RNA transcripts. *Molecular and cellular biology, 28*(17), 5446–5457.

C58.   Falk, S., Bonneau, F., Ebert, J., Kögel, A., & Conti, E. (2017). Mpp6 incorporation in the nuclear exosome contributes to RNA channeling through the Mtr4 helicase. *Cell reports, 20*(10), 2279–2286.

C59.   Cheng, Q., Wang, W., Liu, J., Lv, Z., Ji, W., Yu, J., ... & Yang, Y. (2023). Elevated MPP6 expression correlates with an unfavorable prognosis, angiogenesis and immune evasion in hepatocellular carcinoma. *Frontiers in Immunology, 14*, 1173848.

C60.   Wang, H. Y., Lin, W., Dyck, J. A., Yeakley, J. M., Songyang, Z., Cantley, L. C., & Fu, X. D. (1998). SRPK2: a differentially expressed SR protein-specific kinase involved in mediating the interaction and localization of pre-mRNA splicing factors in mammalian cells. *The Journal of cell biology, 140*(4), 737–750.

C61.   Sridhara, S. C., Carvalho, S., Grosso, A. R., Gallego-Paez, L. M., Carmo-Fonseca, M., & de Almeida, S. F. (2017). Transcription dynamics prevent RNA-mediated genomic instability through SRPK2-dependent DDX23 phosphorylation. *Cell reports, 18*(2), 334–343.

C62.   Wang, G., Sheng, W., Tang, J., Li, X., Zhou, J., & Dong, M. (2020). Cooperation of SRPK2, Numb and p53 in the malignant biology and chemosensitivity of colorectal cancer. *Bioscience Reports, 40*(1), BSR20191488.

C63.   Vreeken, D., Bruikman, C. S., Stam, W., Cox, S. M. L., Nagy, Z., Zhang, H., ... & van Gils, J. M. (2021). Downregulation of endothelial plexin A4 under inflammatory conditions impairs vascular integrity. *Frontiers in Cardiovascular Medicine, 8*, 633609.

C64.   Schulte, E. C., Stahl, I., Czamara, D., Ellwanger, D. C., Eck, S., Graf, E., ... & Winkelmann, J. (2013). Rare variants in PLXNA4 and Parkinson's disease. *PloS one, 8*(11), e79145.

C65.   Kigel, B., Rabinowicz, N., Varshavsky, A., Kessler, O., & Neufeld, G. (2011). Plexin-A4 promotes tumor progression and tumor angiogenesis by enhancement of VEGF and bFGF signaling. *Blood, The Journal of the American Society of Hematology, 118*(15), 4285–4296.

C66.   Gopisetty, G., & Thangarajan, R. (2016). Mammalian mitochondrial ribosomal small subunit (MRPS) genes: A putative role in human disease. *Gene, 589*(1), 27–35.

C67.   Revathi Paramasivam, O., Gopisetty, G., Subramani, J., & Thangarajan, R. (2021). Expression and affinity purification of recombinant mammalian mitochondrial ribosomal small subunit (MRPS) proteins and protein–protein interaction analysis indicate putative role in tumourigenic cellular processes. *The journal of biochemistry, 169*(6), 675–692.

C68.   Gonzalez-Giraldo, Y., Camargo, A., Lopez-Leon, S., Adan, A., & Forero, D. A. (2015). A functional SNP in MIR124-1, a brain expressed miRNA gene, is associated with aggressiveness in a Colombian sample. *European Psychiatry, 30*(4), 499–503.

C69.   Nardone, S., Sams, D. S., Zito, A., Reuveni, E., & Elliott, E. (2017). Dysregulation of cortical neuron DNA methylation profile in autism spectrum disorder. *Cerebral Cortex, 27*(12), 5739–5754.

C70. Svahn, A. J., Giacomotto, J., Graeber, M. B., Rinkwitz, S., & Becker, T. S. (2016). miR-124 Contributes to the functional maturity of microglia. *Developmental neurobiology, 76*(5), 507–518.

C71. Liu, Y., Yang, Y., Wang, X., Yin, S., Liang, B., Zhang, Y., ... & Zhang, Q. (2023). Function of microRNA-124 in the Pathogenesis of Cancer. *International journal of oncology, 64*(1), 6.

C72. Moskovitz, J., Bar-Noy, S., Williams, W. M., Requena, J., Berlett, B. S., & Stadtman, E. R. (2001). Methionine sulfoxide reductase (MsrA) is a regulator of antioxidant defense and lifespan in mammals. *Proceedings of the National Academy of Sciences, 98*(23), 12920–12925.

C73. De Luca, A., Sanna, F., Sallese, M., Ruggiero, C., Grossi, M., Sacchetta, P., ... & Favaloro, B. (2010). Methionine sulfoxide reductase A down-regulation in human breast cancer cells results in a more aggressive phenotype. *Proceedings of the National Academy of Sciences, 107*(43), 18628–18633.

C74. Ransohoff, J. D., Wei, Y., & Khavari, P. A. (2018). The functions and unique features of long intergenic non-coding RNA. *Nature reviews. Molecular cell biology, 19*(3), 143–157.

C75. Karolchik, D., Hinrichs, A. S., Furey, T. S., Roskin, K. M., Sugnet, C. W., Haussler, D., & Kent, W. J. (2004). The UCSC Table Browser data retrieval tool. *Nucleic acids research, 32*(suppl_1), D493-D496.

C76. Vahidnezhad, H., Youssefian, L., Harvey, N., Tavasoli, A. R., Saeidian, A. H., Sotoudeh, S., ... & Uitto, J. (2022). Mutation update: The spectra of PLEC sequence variants and related plectinopathies. *Human Mutation, 43*(12), 1706–1731.

C77. Potokar, M., & Jorgačevski, J. (2021). Plectin in the central nervous system and a putative role in brain astrocytes. *Cells, 10*(9), 2353.

C78. Paumard-Hernández, B., Calvete, O., Inglada Pérez, L., Tejero, H., Al-Shahrour, F., Pita, G., ... & Benítez, J. (2018). Whole exome sequencing identifies PLEC, EXO5 and DNAH7 as novel susceptibility genes in testicular cancer. *International journal of cancer, 143*(8), 1954–1962.

C79. Wang, Y., Yu, Y., Pang, Y., Yu, H., Zhang, W., Zhao, X., & Yu, J. (2021). The distinct roles of zinc finger CCHC-type (ZCCHC) superfamily proteins in the regulation of RNA metabolism. *RNA biology, 18*(12), 2107–2126.

C80. Pakhomova, T., Moshareva, M., Vasilkova, D., Zatsepin, T., Dontsova, O., & Rubtsova, M. (2022). Role of RNA biogenesis factors in the processing and transport of human telomerase RNA. *Biomedicines, 10*(6), 1275.

C81.   Leeman-Neill, R. J., Song, D., Bizarro, J., Wacheul, L., Rothschild, G., Singh, S., ... & Basu, U. (2023). Noncoding mutations cause super-enhancer retargeting resulting in protein synthesis dysregulation during B cell lymphoma progression. *Nature genetics, 55*(12), 2160–2174.

C82.   Bhattacharya, R., & Cabral, F. (2004). A ubiquitous β-tubulin disrupts microtubule assembly and inhibits cell proliferation. *Molecular biology of the cell, 15*(7), 3123–3131.

C83.   Zhang, W., Bojorquez-Gomez, A., Velez, D. O., Xu, G., Sanchez, K. S., Shen, J. P., ... & Ideker, T. (2018). A global transcriptional network connecting noncoding mutations to changes in tumor gene expression. *Nature genetics, 50*(4), 613–620.

C84.   Liu, F., Gong, X., Yao, X., Cui, L., Yin, Z., Li, C., ... & Wang, F. (2019). Variation in the CACNB2 gene is associated with functional connectivity of the Hippocampus in bipolar disorder. *BMC psychiatry, 19*, 1–7.

C85.   Yoon, S., Piguel, N. H., & Penzes, P. (2022). Roles and mechanisms of ankyrin-G in neuropsychiatric disorders. *Experimental & Molecular Medicine, 54*(7), 867–877.

C86.   Tang, L., Liu, J., Zhu, Y., Duan, J., Chen, Y., Wei, Y., ... & Tang, Y. (2021). ANK3 gene polymorphism Rs10994336 influences executive functions by modulating methylation in patients with bipolar disorder. *Frontiers in Neuroscience, 15*, 682873.

C87.   Tan, Y., Meng, W., Jiang, Z., Li, N., Zhang, T., Zhang, J., ... & Guan, Y. (2024). A comprehensive analysis of the prognostic and immunological role of ANK3 in pan-cancer. *Translational Cancer Research, 13*(2).

C88.   Wang, Y., Shin, I., Li, J., & Liu, A. (2021). Crystal structure of human cysteamine dioxygenase provides a structural rationale for its function as an oxygen sensor. *Journal of Biological Chemistry, 297*(4).

C89.   Sarkar, B., Kulharia, M., & Mantha, A. K. (2017). Understanding human thiol dioxygenase enzymes: structure to function, and biology to pathology. *International journal of experimental pathology, 98*(2), 52–66.

C90. Shen, D., Tian, L., Yang, F., Li, J., Li, X., Yao, Y., ... & Wang, R. (2021). ADO/hypotaurine: a novel metabolic pathway contributing to glioblastoma development. *Cell death discovery*, *7*(1), 21.

C91. Kiang, K. M. Y., Zhang, P., Li, N., Zhu, Z., Jin, L., & Leung, G. K. K. (2020). Loss of cytoskeleton protein ADD3 promotes tumor growth and angiogenesis in glioblastoma multiforme. *Cancer letters*, *474*, 118–126.

C92. Reynolds, L. M., Howard, T. D., Ruczinski, I., Kanchan, K., Seeds, M. C., Mathias, R. A., & Chilton, F. H. (2018). Tissue-specific impact of FADS cluster variants on FADS1 and FADS2 gene expression. *PloS one*, *13*(3), e0194610.

C93. Koletzko, B., Reischl, E., Tanjung, C., Gonzalez-Casanova, I., Ramakrishnan, U., Meldrum, S., ... & Demmelmair, H. (2019). FADS1 and FADS2 polymorphisms modulate fatty acid metabolism and dietary impact on health. *Annual review of nutrition*, *39*(1), 21–44.

C94. Zhao, T., Gao, P., Li, Y., Tian, H., Ma, D., Sun, N., ... & Qi, X. (2023). Investigating the role of FADS family members in breast cancer based on bioinformatic analysis and experimental validation. *Frontiers in Immunology, 14*, 1074242.

C95. Hoefner, C., Bryde, T. H., Pihl, C., Tiedemann, S. N., Bresson, S. E., Hotiana, H. A., ... & Marzec, M. T. (2023). FK506-binding protein 2 participates in proinsulin folding. *Biomolecules*, *13*(1), 152.

C96. Sun, Z., Qin, X., Fang, J., Tang, Y., & Fan, Y. (2021). Multi-omics analysis of the expression and prognosis for FKBP gene family in renal cancer. *Frontiers in Oncology*, *11*, 697534.

C97. Schuurs-Hoeijmakers, J. H., Oh, E. C., Vissers, L. E., Swinkels, M. E., Gilissen, C., Willemsen, M. A., ... & Brunner, H. G. (2012). Recurrent de novo mutations in PACS1 cause defective cranial-neural-crest migration and define a recognizable intellectual-disability syndrome. *The American Journal of Human Genetics*, *91*(6), 1122–1127.

C98. Jitrapakdee, S., & Wallace, J. C. (1999). Structure, function and regulation of pyruvate carboxylase. *Biochemical Journal*, *340*(1), 1–16.

C99. Jitrapakdee, S., Vidal-Puig, A., & Wallace, J. C. (2006). Anaplerotic roles of pyruvate carboxylase in mammalian tissues. *Cellular and Molecular Life Sciences CMLS*, *63*, 843–854.

C100. Kiesel, V. A., Sheeley, M. P., Coleman, M. F., Cotul, E. K., Donkin, S. S., Hursting, S. D., ... & Teegarden, D. (2021). Pyruvate carboxylase and cancer progression. *Cancer & metabolism, 9*(1), 20.

C101. Caumes, R., Smol, T., Thuillier, C., Balerdi, M., Lestienne-Roche, C., Manouvrier-Hanu, S., & Ghoumid, J. (2020). Phenotypic spectrum of SHANK2-related neurodevelopmental disorder. *European Journal of Medical Genetics, 63*(12), 104072.

C102. Guilmatre, A., Huguet, G., Delorme, R., & Bourgeron, T. (2014). The emerging role of SHANK genes in neuropsychiatric disorders. *Developmental neurobiology, 74*(2), 113–122.

C103. Pappas, A. L., Bey, A. L., Wang, X., Rossi, M., Kim, Y. H., Yan, H., ... & Jiang, Y. H. (2017). Deficiency of Shank2 causes mania-like behavior that responds to mood stabilizers. *JCI insight, 2*(20), e92052.

C104. Lopez, G., Conkrite, K. L., Doepner, M., Rathi, K. S., Modi, A., Vaksman, Z., ... & Diskin, S. J. (2020). Somatic structural variation targets neurodevelopmental genes and identifies SHANK2 as a tumor suppressor in neuroblastoma. *Genome research, 30*(9), 1228–1242.

C105. Psychiatric GWAS Consortium Bipolar Disorder Working Group (2011). Large-scale genome-wide association analysis of bipolar disorder identifies a new susceptibility locus near ODZ4. *Nature genetics, 43*(10), 977–983.

C106. Tucker, R. P., & Chiquet-Ehrismann, R. (2006). Teneurins: a conserved family of transmembrane proteins involved in intercellular signaling during development. *Developmental biology, 290*(2), 237–245.

C107. Heinrich, A., Lourdusamy, A., Tzschoppe, J., Vollstädt-Klein, S., Bühler, M., Steiner, S., ... & IMAGEN consortium. (2013). The risk variant in ODZ 4 for bipolar disorder impacts on amygdala activation during reward processing. *Bipolar disorders, 15*(4), 440–445.

C108. Ziegler, A., Corvalán, A., Roa, I., Brañes, J. A., & Wollscheid, B. (2012). Teneurin protein family: an emerging role in human tumorigenesis and drug resistance. *Cancer letters, 326*(1), 1–7.

C109. Bhat, S., Dao, D. T., Terrillion, C. E., Arad, M., Smith, R. J., Soldatov, N. M., & Gould, T. D. (2012). CACNA1C (Cav1. 2) in the pathophysiology of psychiatric disease. *Progress in neurobiology*, *99*(1), 1–14.

C110. Datta, D., Yang, S., Joyce, M. K. P., Woo, E., McCarroll, S. A., Gonzalez-Burgos, G., ... & Arnsten, A. F. (2024). Key roles of CACNA1C/Cav1. 2 and CALB1/calbindin in prefrontal neurons altered in cognitive disorders. *JAMA psychiatry*, *81*(9), 870–881.

C111. Hannah, J., & Zhou, P. (2015). Distinct and overlapping functions of the cullin E3 ligase scaffolding proteins CUL4A and CUL4B. *Gene*, *573*(1), 33–45.

C112. Lennon, M. J., Jones, S. P., Lovelace, M. D., Guillemin, G. J., & Brew, B. J. (2017). Bcl11b—a critical neurodevelopmental transcription factor—roles in health and disease. *Frontiers in cellular neuroscience*, *11*, 89.

C113. Holmes, T. D., Pandey, R. V., Helm, E. Y., Schlums, H., Han, H., Campbell, T. M., ... & Bryceson, Y. T. (2021). The transcription factor Bcl11b promotes both canonical and adaptive NK cell differentiation. *Frontiers in cellular neuroscience*, *6*(57), eabc9801.

C114. Kranz, T. M., Ekawardhani, S., Lin, M. K., Witzmann, S. R., Streit, F., Schuelter, U., ... & Meyer, J. (2012). The chromosome 15q14 locus for bipolar disorder and schizophrenia: is C15orf53 a major candidate gene?. *Journal of psychiatric research*, *46*(11), 1414–1420.

C115. Wang, J. C., Foroud, T., Hinrichs, A. L., Le, N. X., Bertelsen, S., Budde, J. P., ... & Goate, A. M. (2013). A genome-wide association study of alcohol-dependence symptom counts in extended pedigrees identifies C15orf53. *Molecular psychiatry*, *18*(11), 1218–1224.

C116. Abdou, Y., Baird, A., Dolan, J., Lee, S., & Park, S. (2019). Machine learning-assisted prognostication based on genomic expression in the tumour microenvironment of estrogen receptor positive and her2 negative breast cancer. *Annals of Oncology*, *30*, 55–56.

C117. Okamoto, N., Tsuchiya, Y., Miya, F., Tsunoda, T., Yamashita, K., Boroevich, K. A., ... & Kitagawa, D. (2017). A novel genetic syndrome with STARD9 mutation and abnormal spindle morphology. *American Journal of Medical Genetics Part A*, *173*(10), 2690–2696.

C118. Torres, J. Z., Summers, M. K., Peterson, D., Brauer, M. J., Lee, J., Senese, S., ... & Jackson, P. K. (2011). The STARD9/Kif16a kinesin associates with mitotic microtubules and regulates spindle pole assembly. *Cell, 147*(6), 1309–1323.

C119. Clutario, K. M., & Torres, J. Z. (2019). Proteomic and Functional Characterization of STARD9. *The FASEB Journal, 33*(S1), 475–3.

C120. Shin, D. M., Dehoff, M., Luo, X., Kang, S. H., Tu, J., Nayak, S. K., ... & Muallem, S. (2003). Homer 2 tunes G protein–coupled receptors stimulus intensity by regulating RGS proteins and PLCβ GAP activities. *The Journal of cell biology, 162*(2), 293–303.

C121. Szumlinski, K. K., Lominac, K. D., Oleson, E. B., Walker, J. K., Mason, A., Dehoff, M. H., ... & Kalivas, P. W. (2005). Homer2 is necessary for EtOH-induced neuroplasticity. *Journal of Neuroscience, 25*(30), 7054–7061.

C122. Luo, P., Liang, C., Jing, W., Zhu, M., Zhou, H., Chai, H., ... & Tu, J. (2021). Homer2 and Homer3 act as novel biomarkers in diagnosis of hepatitis B virus-induced hepatocellular carcinoma. *Journal of Cancer, 12*(12), 3439.

C123. Nicolas, E., Poitelon, Y., Chouery, E., Salem, N., Levy, N., Mégarbané, A., & Delague, V. (2010). CAMOS, a nonprogressive, autosomal recessive, congenital cerebellar ataxia, is caused by a mutant zinc-finger protein, ZNF592. *European journal of human genetics, 18*(10), 1107–1113.

C124. Braun, E., & Sauter, D. (2019). Furin-mediated protein processing in infectious diseases and cancer. *Clinical & translational immunology, 8*(8), e1073.

C125. Benslimane, Y., Sánchez-Osuna, M., Coulombe-Huntington, J., Bertomeu, T., Henry, D., Huard, C., ... & Harrington, L. (2021). A novel p53 regulator, C16ORF72/TAPR1, buffers against telomerase inhibition. *Aging Cell, 20*(4), e13331.

C126. Amici, D. R., Ansel, D. J., Metz, K. A., Smith, R. S., Phoumyvong, C. M., Gayatri, S., ... & Mendillo, M. L. (2022). C16orf72/HAPSTR1 is a molecular rheostat in an integrated network of stress response pathways. *Proceedings of the National Academy of Sciences, 119*(27), e2111262119.

C127. Strehlow, V., Heyne, H. O., Vlaskamp, D. R., Marwick, K. F., Rudolf, G., De Bellescize, J., ... & Lemke, J. R. (2019). GRIN2A-related disorders: genotype and functional consequence predict phenotype. *Brain, 142*(1), 80–92.

C128. Endele, S., Rosenberger, G., Geider, K., Popp, B., Tamer, C., Stefanova, I., ... & Kutsche, K. (2010). Mutations in GRIN2A and

GRIN2B encoding regulatory subunits of NMDA receptors cause variable neurodevelopmental phenotypes. *Nature genetics, 42*(11), 1021–1026.

C129. Costantini, A., Alm, J. J., Tonelli, F., Valta, H., Huber, C., Tran, A. N., ... & Mäkitie, O. (2020). Novel RPL13 variants and variable clinical expressivity in a human ribosomopathy with spondyloepimetaphyseal dysplasia. *Journal of Bone and Mineral Research, 36*(2), 283–297.

C130. Kardos, G. R., Dai, M. S., & Robertson, G. P. (2014). Growth inhibitory effects of large subunit ribosomal proteins in melanoma. *Pigment cell & melanoma research, 27*(5), 801–812.

C131. Wills, Z. P., Mandel-Brehm, C., Mardinly, A. R., McCord, A. E., Giger, R. J., & Greenberg, M. E. (2012). The nogo receptor family restricts synapse number in the developing hippocampus. *Neuron, 73*(3), 466–481.

C132. Pathak, G. P., Shah, R., Kennedy, B. E., Murphy, J. P., Clements, D., Konda, P., ... & Gujar, S. (2018). RTN4 knockdown dysregulates the AKT pathway, destabilizes the cytoskeleton, and enhances paclitaxel-induced cytotoxicity in cancers. *Molecular Therapy, 26*(8), 2019–2033.

C133. Garratt, A. N., Özcelik, C., & Birchmeier, C. (2003). ErbB2 pathways in heart and neural diseases. *Trends in Cardiovascular Medicine, 13*(2), 80–86.

C134. Harari, D., & Yarden, Y. (2000). Molecular mechanisms underlying ErbB2/HER2 action in breast cancer. *Oncogene, 19*(53), 6102–6114.

C135. Agis-Balboa, R. C., Pavelka, Z., Kerimoglu, C., & Fischer, A. (2013). Loss of HDAC5 impairs memory function: implications for Alzheimer's disease. *Journal of Alzheimer's Disease, 33*(1), 35–44.

C136. Peixoto, P., Castronovo, V., Matheus, N., Polese, C., Peulen, O., Gonzalez, A., ... & Mottet, D. (2012). HDAC5 is required for maintenance of pericentric heterochromatin, and controls cell-cycle progression and survival of human cancer cells. *Cell Death & Differentiation, 19*(7), 1239–1252.

C137. Li, W., Xiao, J., Zhou, X., Xu, M., Hu, C., Xu, X., ... & Wang, H. (2015). STK4 regulates TLR pathways and protects against chronic inflammation–related hepatocellular carcinoma. *The Journal of clinical investigation, 125*(11), 4239–4254.

C138. Abdollahpour, H., Appaswamy, G., Kotlarz, D., Diestelhorst, J., Beier, R., Schäffer, A. A., ... & Klein, C. (2012). The phenotype of human STK4 deficiency. *Blood, The Journal of the American Society of Hematology, 119*(15), 3450–3457.

C139. Clauss, A., Lilja, H., & Lundwall, Å. (2005). The evolution of a genetic locus encoding small serine proteinase inhibitors. *Biochemical and biophysical research communications, 333*(2), 383–389.

C140. Bortolami, A., Yu, W., Forzisi, E., Ercan, K., Kadakia, R., Murugan, M., ... & Sesti, F. (2023). Integrin-KCNB1 potassium channel complexes regulate neocortical neuronal development and are implicated in epilepsy. *Cell Death & Differentiation, 30*(3), 687–701.

C141. Koh, Y. I., Oh, K. S., Kim, J. A., Noh, B., Choi, H. J., Joo, S. Y., ... & Gee, H. Y. (2022). OSBPL2 mutations impair autophagy and lead to hearing loss, potentially remedied by rapamycin. *Autophagy, 18*(11), 2593–2614.

C142. Pietrangelo, A., & Ridgway, N. D. (2018). Golgi localization of oxysterol binding protein-related protein 4L (ORP4L) is regulated by ligand binding. *Journal of Cell Science, 131*(14), jcs215335.

C143. Tian, K., Ying, Y., Huang, J., Wu, H., Wei, C., Li, L., ... & Wu, L. (2023). The expression, immune infiltration, prognosis, and experimental validation of OSBPL family genes in liver cancer. *BMC cancer, 23*(1), 244.

C144. Palmieri, F. (2014). Mitochondrial transporters of the SLC25 family and associated diseases: a review. *Journal of inherited metabolic disease, 37*, 565–575.

C145. Agrimi, G., Russo, A., Scarcia, P., & Palmieri, F. (2012). The human gene SLC25A17 encodes a peroxisomal transporter of coenzyme A, FAD and NAD+. *Biochemical Journal, 443*(1), 241–247.

C146. Zhou, H., Li, J., He, Y., Xia, X., Liu, J., & Xiong, H. (2024). SLC25A17 inhibits autophagy to promote triple-negative breast cancer tumorigenesis by ROS-mediated JAK2/STAT3 signaling pathway. *Cancer Cell International, 24*(1), 85.

APPENDIX D

A List of Scientific Journals Consulted

1. *Acta Neurologica Scandinavica*
2. *Acta Psychiatrica Belgica*
3. *Acta Psychiatrica Scandinavica*
4. *Actas Espanolas de Psiquiatria*
5. *Advances in Medical Biochemistry, Genomics, Physiology, and Pathology*
6. *Advances in Psychiatric Treatment*
7. *Agency for Healthcare Research and Quality (USA)*
8. *Aggression and Violent Behavior*
9. *Aging*
10. *Aging Cell*
11. *The American Journal of Human Genetics*
12. *American Journal of Medical Genetics Part A*
13. *The American Journal of Medicine*
14. *American Journal of Physiology-Cell Physiology*
15. *The American Journal of Psychiatry*
16. *American Journal of Translational Research*
17. *American Psychiatric Press*
18. *American Psychologist*
19. *American Scientist*
20. *Angewandte Chemie (International ed. in English)*
21. *Annals of Clinical and Translational Neurology*
22. *Annals of Neurology*
23. *Annals of Oncology*
24. *Annals of Saudi Medicine*
25. *Annals of the New York Academy of Sciences*

26. *Annual APS Meeting: Research Abstracts*
27. *Annual Review of Biochemistry*
28. *Annual Review of Nutrition*
29. *Annual Review of Physiology*
30. *Antioxidants & Redox Signaling*
31. *Autophagy*
32. *Archives of General Psychiatry*
33. *Archives of Neuropsychiatry*
34. *Biochemical and Biophysical Research Communications*
35. *Biochemical Journal*
36. *Biochemistry*
37. *Biochimie*
38. *Biological Psychiatry*
39. *Biological Research*
40. *Biology*
41. *Biomedical Reports*
42. *Biomedicines*
43. *Biomolecules*
44. *Biophysical Journal*
45. *bioRxiv*
46. *Bioscience Reports*
47. *BioTech*
48. *Bipolar Disorders*
49. *Bipolar Disorders: Basic Mechanisms and Therapeutic Implications*
50. *Blood*
51. *Blood Cells, Molecules, and Diseases*
52. *BMC Cancer*
53. *BMC Psychiatry*
54. *Brain*
55. *Brain Structure and Function*
56. *Brazilian Journal of Psychiatry*
57. *British Journal of Psychiatry*
58. *Bulletin de l'Académie Nationale de Médecine*
59. *Bulletin of Experimental Biology and Medicine*
60. *Cancer & Metabolism*
61. *Cancer Cell International*
62. *Cancer Drug Resistance*
63. *Cancer Letters*
64. *Cancer Research*

103. *European Journal of Medical Genetics*
104. *European Journal of Medicinal Chemistry*
105. *European Journal of Pharmaceutical Sciences*
106. *European Journal of Pharmacology*
107. *European Molecular Biology Organization Journal*
108. *European Molecular Biology Organization Reports*
109. *European Psychiatry*
110. *Experimental & Molecular Medicine*
111. *Experimental Neurology*
112. *The FASEB Journal*
113. *Federation of American Societies for Experimental Biology Journal*
114. *Fluids and Barriers of the CNS*
115. *Focus: Journal of Life Long Learning in Psychiatry*
116. *Free Radical Biology and Medicine*
117. *Frontiers in Bioscience*
118. *Frontiers in Cardiovascular Medicine*
119. *Frontiers in Cellular Neuroscience*
120. *Frontiers in Genetics*
121. *Frontiers in Immunology*
122. *Frontiers in Molecular Biosciences*
123. *Frontiers in Neurology*
124. *Frontiers in Neuroscience*
125. *Frontiers in Oncology*
126. *Frontiers in Physiology*
127. *Frontiers in Psychiatry*
128. *Gene*
129. *Gene Expression*
130. *Genes, Brain and Behavior*
131. *Genetic Engineering and Biotechnology News*
132. *Genome Biology*
133. *Genome Research*
134. *Harvard Review of Psychiatry*
135. *Heredity*
136. *Historical Studies in the Physical and Biological Sciences.*
137. *Human Brain Mapping*
138. *Human Genetics*
139. *Human Molecular Genetics*
140. *Human Mutation*
141. *International Journal of Biological Sciences*

142. *International Journal of Bipolar Disorders*
143. *International Journal of Cancer*
144. *International Journal of Experimental Pathology*
145. *International Journal of Health Sciences*
146. *International Journal of Molecular Medicine*
147. *International Journal of Molecular Sciences*
148. *International Journal of Neuropsychopharmacology*
149. *International Journal of Neuroscience*
150. *International Journal of Oncology*
151. *International Scholarly Research Notices*
152. *JAMA Neurology*
153. *JAMA Psychiatry*
154. *Journal of Affective Disorders*
155. *Journal of Alzheimer's Disease*
156. *The Journal of Anatomy*
157. *Journal of Biochemistry*
158. *Journal of Biological Chemistry*
159. *Journal of Bone and Mineral Research*
160. *Journal of Cancer*
161. *Journal of Cell Biology*
162. *Journal of Cell Science*
163. *Journal of Cerebral Blood Flow & Metabolism*
164. *Journal of Chemical Education*
165. *The Journal of Clinical Investigation*
166. *Journal of Clinical Investigation Insight*
167. *Journal of Clinical Neurophysiology*
168. *Journal of Clinical Neuroscience*
169. *Journal of Clinical Psychiatry*
170. *Journal of General Physiology*
171. *Journal of Human Hypertension*
172. *The Journal of Immunology*
173. *Journal of Immunology Research*
174. *Journal of Inherited Metabolic Disease*
175. *Journal of Medical Genetics*
176. *Journal of Mental Health*
177. *Journal of Microscopy and Ultrastructure*
178. *Journal of Molecular Cell Biology*
179. *Journal of Neuroimmune Pharmacology*
180. *Journal of Neuropathology & Experimental Neurology*

181. *Journal of Neuroscience*
182. *Journal of Physiological Sciences*
183. *Journal of Physiology*
184. *Journal of Psychiatric Research*
185. *Journal of Psychiatry and Neuroscience*
186. *Journal of Trace Elements in Medicine and Biology*
187. *Journal of Translational Genetics and Genomics*
188. *Journal of Translational Medicine*
189. *Journal of Zhejiang University SCIENCE B*
190. *The Lancet*
191. *The Lancet Neurology*
192. *The Lancet Psychiatry*
193. *Medical Journal of Australia*
194. *Medicinal Research Reviews*
195. *Metallothionein IV*
196. *Methods*
197. *MIND*
198. *Molecular and Cellular Biology*
199. *Molecular Biology of the Cell*
200. *Molecular Biology Reports*
201. *Molecular Cell*
202. *Molecular Genetics & Genomic Medicine*
203. *Molecular Medicine Reports*
204. *Molecular Neurobiology*
205. *Molecular Psychiatry*
206. *Molecular Therapy*
207. *Monitor on Psychology*
208. *Mutation Research-Reviews in Mutation Research*
209. *Nature*
210. *Nature Biotechnology*
211. *Nature Communications*
212. *Nature Education*
213. *Nature Genetics*
214. *Nature Methods*
215. *Nature Neuroscience*
216. *Nature Reviews Cancer*
217. *Nature Reviews Disease Primers*
218. *Nature Reviews Immunology*
219. *Nature Reviews Molecular Cell Biology*

220. *Nature Reviews Neuroscience*
221. *Neurobiology of Disease*
222. *Neurochemical Research*
223. *Neurochemistry International*
224. *Neuroglia*
225. *Neuroinflammation*
226. *Neurology*
227. *Neuron*
228. *The Neuron: Cell and Molecular Biology*
229. *Neuropsychiatric Disease and Treatment*
230. *Neuropsychopharmacology*
231. *Neuroscience*
232. *The Neuroscientist*
233. *Neuroscience & Biobehavioral Reviews*
234. *Neuroscience Research*
235. *The Neuroscientist*
236. *Neurotoxicity Research*
237. *Nöropsikiyatri Arşivi*
238. *Nucleic Acids Research*
239. *Nutrition*
240. *Oncogene*
241. *OncoTargets and Therapy*
242. *Origins of Life and Evolution of the Biosphere*
243. *Pflügers Archiv: European Journal of Physiology*
244. *Pharmacogenomics*
245. *Photochemistry and photobiology*
246. *Physical Review*
247. *Physiological Reviews*
248. *Pigment Cell & Melanoma Research*
249. *PLOS One*
250. *Practical Neurology*
251. *Proceedings of the National Academy of Sciences*
252. *Proceedings of the Royal Society B: Biological Sciences*
253. *Progress in Neurobiology*
254. *Progress in Neuro-Psychopharmacology & Biological Psychiatry*
255. *Psychiatric Clinics of North America*
256. *Psychiatric Genetics*
257. *Psychiatry and Clinical Neurosciences*
258. *Psychiatry Investigation*

259. *Psychiatry Research*
260. *Psychoneuroendocrinology*
261. *Psychopharmacology and Biological Psychiatry*
262. *Psychosocial Rehabilitation Journal*
263. *Reviews in Mutation Research*
264. *Reviews of Modern Physics*
265. *RNA Biology*
266. *Schizophrenia Bulletin*
267. *Schizophrenia Research*
268. *Science*
269. *Science Immunology*
270. *Science Translational Medicine*
271. *Scientific American*
272. *Scientific Reports*
273. *Signal Transduction and Targeted Therapy*
274. *Singapore Medical Journal*
275. *Springer*
276. *Tohoku Journal of Experimental Medicine*
277. *Toxicologic Pathology*
278. *Translational Cancer Research*
279. *Translational Psychiatry*
280. *Trends in Cardiovascular Medicine*
281. *Trends in Cell Biology*
282. *Trends in Neuroscience*
283. *Trends in Pharmacological Sciences*
284. *World Journal of Gastroenterology*
285. *World Psychiatry*
286. *Yale Journal of Biology and Medicine*
287. *Yearbook of Intensive Care and Emergency Medicine 1998*

Glossary

5-HT$_{1A}$ receptor: In the brain, a G-coupled protein receptor that has a key role in serotonin neurotransmission and also modulates behavior of other neurotransmitters.

8-oxo-dG (8-Oxo-2'-deoxyguanosine): A marker for accelerated DNA damage and elevated oxidative stress. This molecule is formed when DNA guanine is oxidized.

8-oxoguanine DNA glycosylase (OGG1): A key enzyme in base excision repair and a marker for DNA damage and oxidative stress.

Acetyl coenzyme A: An important molecule in metabolism that is involved in many biochemical reactions. It is the primary source of acetyl groups for epigenetic histone modification, synthesis of the neurotransmitter acetylcholine, and fat metabolism.

Acetyl group: In organic chemistry, a functional group with the chemical formula COCH$_3$. The acetyl group consists of a methyl group single-bonded to a carbonyl.

Acetylcholine: A monoamine neurotransmitter essential to memory, communication between nerves and muscles, and parasympathetic activity.

Acetyltransferase: An enzyme that transfers an acetyl group to a histone of another protein.

Action potential: Also known as a neuron firing event, the brief reversal of electric potential (voltage) of a neuron membrane that can eject neurotransmitters into a synapse.

Adduct: In microbiology, a foreign chemical molecule that has bonded to a segment of DNA, altering its structure and potentially leading to mutations.

Adenosine triphosphate (ATP): A compound consisting of an adenosine molecule bonded to three phosphate groups that are present in all living tissue and is the cell's primary energy source.

Adenosine: In biology, a purine nucleoside composed of adenine attached to a ribose sugar molecule. It serves as a building block of RNA and a precursor to ATP.

ADHD: See *Attention-deficit/hyperactivity disorder.*

AIS: See *Axon initial segment.*

ALC1 (also known as CHD1L): A chromatin-remodeling enzyme required for efficient base excision repair.

Allele: An expression used to describe an alternative form or version of a gene. A person inherits one allele from each autosomal gene from each parent.

ALS: A progressive neurodegenerative disease that affects nerve cells in the brain and spinal cord.

Alternative splicing: A process in which a single gene may express several different proteins during transcription by various mechanisms, including inclusion of an intron or abnormal positioning of an exon.

Alzheimer's disease: A progressive, degenerative brain disease that destroys brain cells, causing memory loss and problems with thinking and behavior.

Amino acids: Molecules containing an amine group, a carboxylic acid and a side chain that serve as building blocks for proteins, neurotransmitters, and hormones.

Amoeba: A tiny, single-celled organism commonly found in water that moves and feeds by extending temporary projections called pseudopodia (false feet).

Amphetamine: A central nervous system stimulant drug known to produce increased wakefulness and focus. Amphetamines are believed to act by increasing levels of dopamine and norepinephrine in the brain.

Amygdala: An almond-shaped structure located deep within the medial temporal lobes of the brain that are essential to memory and emotional reaction.

Amyotrophic lateral sclerosis (ALS): A progressive neurodegenerative disease that affects nerve cells in the brain and spinal cord.

Angelman syndrome: A rare genetic disorder involving developmental delays, disabilities, and speech impairments due to loss of function of the UBE3A gene.

Angiogenesis: The physiological process involving the growth of new blood vessels from pre-existing vessels.

Anhedonia: A psychological term that refers to the inability or reduced capacity to experience pleasure or enjoyment from activities that are typically rewarding.

Antagomirs: A class of chemically engineered oligonucleotides designed to silence endogenous microRNAs.

Anticonvulsants: A class of drugs used to reduce or prevent epilepsy and seizures.

Antidepressant: A psychiatric medication used to alleviate mood disorders, such as major depression, dysthymia, and anxiety disorders. This family of drugs includes monoamine oxidase inhibitors, tricyclic antidepressants, SSRIs, and SNRIs.

Antioxidant: An atom, molecule, or other substance which protects cells from damage caused by free radicals.

Anxiety: A mental condition characterized by irrational or inappropriate expressions of fear.

APOE (Apolipoprotein E): A class of proteins essential for the normal catabolism of triglyceride-rich lipoprotein constituents. Genetic APOE mutations have been associated with higher risk of Alzheimer's disease.

Apoenzyme: A genetically expressed protein that requires the addition of an atom, molecule, or ion before it can function as an effective enzyme.

Apoptosis: A mechanism of cell death that may be genetically programmed or caused by an environmental insult.

Arginine: A basic amino acid that is a constituent of most proteins.

Arginine residue: An arginine molecule that has been incorporated into a protein or peptide chain.

ASD: See *Autism spectrum disorder.*

Astrocyte: A star-shaped glial cell that plays a major role in the support and function of neurons.

Astrocyte end-feet: In biology, flattened astrocyte projections that wrap around brain blood vessels that regulate blood flow, nutrient intake, and waste clearance, as well as enable transport of K+ and other ions.

ATM (ataxia telangiectasia mutated) proteins: Proteins that play a crucial role in responding to DNA double-strand breaks by coordinating repair processes, promoting cell survival, or triggering programmed cell death.

ATP: See *Adenosine triphosphate.*

Attention-deficit/hyperactivity disorder (ADHD): A serious neurobehavioral disorder characterized by persistent symptoms of inattention, hyperactivity, or impulsivity that can be a barrier to academic and career success.

Atypical medications: Also called 2nd generation antipsychotics, a group of tranquilizing drugs used to treat psychiatric conditions including schizophrenia, mania, and bipolar disorder.

Autism spectrum disorder (ASD): A severe disorder of neural development characterized by impaired social interaction and communication, and by restricted and repetitive behaviors.

Autoreceptor: A type of neurotransmitter receptor found on a presynaptic neuron's cell membrane that leads to negative feedback in the presynaptic neuron.

Axon: A long, slender projection of a nerve cell, or neuron that conducts electrical impulses away from the neuron's cell body or "soma."

Axon hillock: A swelling of the axon where it meets the soma.

Axon initial segment (AIS): An axon compartment adjacent to the hillock that sums receptor voltage inputs and generates an action potential when the voltage threshold is reached.

Axon terminal: A specialized region at the end of an axon that contains neurotransmitters that may be released into a synapse.

Base excision repair (BER): An important DNA repair pathway that removes and replaces damaged or inappropriate DNA bases.

BBB: See *Blood-brain barrier*.

BDNF: See *Brain-derived neurotropic factor*.

Benzodiazepine: A class of psychoactive drugs whose core chemical structure is the fusion of a benzene ring and a diazepine ring. Benzodiazepines enhance the effect of the neurotransmitter GABA, which generally results in sedation, reduced anxiety, and improved ability to sleep.

Bidirectional excision: A process where damaged DNA is cut and removed from both sides, leaving a gap that can be filled in with new DNA during the repair process.

Bilayer membrane: A thin polar membrane made of two layers of lipid molecules that form a continuous barrier around cells.

Biochemical: An atom or molecule that participates in chemical processes in the body. There are a vast number of biochemicals in humans, including proteins, enzymes, nutrients, fatty acids, and hormones.

Biochemical individuality: The concept that the nutritional and chemical make-up of each person is unique and that dietary and medical needs therefore vary from person to person.

Biochemical therapy: Medical treatments that use natural body chemicals rather than drugs.

Biotype: A group of people who share specific biochemical factors.

Bipolar disorder: A serious psychiatric condition that usually involves epi-sodes of abnormally elevated energy, cognition, and mood (mania) followed by episodes of clinical depression. The disorder has been subdivided into bipolar 1, bipolar 2, cyclothymia, and other types, based on the nature and severity of mood episodes experienced.

Bipolar disorder with mixed features (also known as mixed states): A form of bipolar disorder that involves simultaneous symptoms of mania and depression.

Bipolar 1 disorder: A type of bipolar disorder involving alternating episodes of severe mania episodes and clinical depression.

Bipolar 2 disorder: A type of bipolar disorder involving mild mania episodes (hypomania) that alternate with periods of severe depression.

Bipolar switching: The transitions between mania and depression that are characteristic of bipolar disorder.

Blood-brain barrier (BBB): High-density cells attached to blood vessels that prevent or restrict the passage of certain chemicals into the brain.

Bookmarking: In biology, regulation of gene expression kinetics by methyl, acetyl or other chemical groups that bind to specific DNA or histone sites. Methyl bookmarks attached to DNA during gestation tend to be permanent regulators of protein expression in cells throughout life and impact physical and mental functioning.

Brain-derived neurotropic factor (BDNF): A protein that is a part of the growth factor family known as neurotrophins. It helps neurons by supporting growth and differentiation through neurogenesis. BDNF dysregulation has been linked with schizophrenia and Alzheimer's disease.

BRCA genes: Two DNA repair genes whose mutations are associated with breast cancer.

Bromodomain: An approximately 110 amino acid protein domain in certain transcription factors that recognize acetylated histones that are available for protein expression. Epigenetic bromodomain therapies are under commercial development for altering expression rates of specific genes. Dysfunction of this domain has been linked to various cancers.

c-Jun N-terminal kinase (JNK): A protein kinase involved in various cellular processes, including cell growth, inflammation, and programmed cell death.

Calcium: Chemical element with symbol Ca and atomic number 20. Calcium is the most abundant mineral in the body.

cAMP: See *Cyclic adenosine monophosphate.*

Cancer: A group of diseases characterized by the uncontrolled growth and spread of abnormal cells.

Canonical: In molecular biology, the most common sequence of amino acids or nucleotides in a DNA or RNA strand. Noncanonical sites are often referred to as mutations or variants.

Capacitor: A device or biochemical system for storing electrical charge. The capacitance of a neuron's bilayer membrane provides the impetus for action potentials.

Catalase: An antioxidant enzyme that catalyzes the decomposition of hydrogen peroxide to water and oxygen.

Catatonia: A symptom of severe mental disorders characterized by stupor, mutism, negativism, rigidity, purposeless excitement, and inappropriate or bizarre posturing.

Caudal projections: In raphe nuclei, projections that pass through the spinal cord and brainstem while other raphe nuclei project to higher brain areas.

Cell type: One of approximately 200 specialized cell groups in humans that perform unique functional roles in the body. Each type has a different structure, size, shape, and organelles.

Cerebellum: A region of the brain that has the appearance of a separate structure beneath the hemispheres. It plays an important role in motor control, the ability to have smooth physical movements, and cognitive functions such as attention and language.

Channelopathy: A disease caused by disturbed function of ion channels or the proteins that regulate them.

Cholinergic: An adjective used to describe enhancement of acetylcholine activity in the brain and the peripheral nervous system.

Chromatin readers: Proteins that recognize specific modifications in DNA and histones that may alter transcription, DNA repair, and other biological processes.

Chromatin: A complex of DNA and histones that package DNA into a small volume to fit in the nucleus, allow mitosis and meiosis, and regulate gene expression and DNA replication.

Chromosome: A cellular structure containing genes that carry instructions for various traits and functions of an organism.

Closed system: In thermodynamics, a system in which heat and work may be exchanged but matter cannot pass through the system's boundary.

Codon: A sequence of three nucleotides in DNA or RNA that code for a specific amino acid.

Coenzyme: A small organic molecule that links to an enzyme, and whose presence is essential to the activity of that enzyme.

Cofactor: A non-protein chemical that is loosely bound to a protein (or enzyme) and enhances the protein's biological activity.

Computational function of neurons: The process of summing voltage inputs from receptors to determine the distance to the threshold voltage for neuron firing.

Conformational: An alteration of the shape of a protein due to temperature change, binding of a molecule, or other factors.

Controlled study: A clinical study that compares people getting treatment (treatment group) to people who do not receive this treatment (control group).

Copy number variations (CNVs): A change in the number of copies of a DNA segment in an individual's genome that may be caused by insertions, deletions, or duplications.

Cortex (or cerebrum): The largest part of the human brain which is associated with higher brain functions such as thought and action. The cerebral cortex is divided into four sections: the frontal lobe, parietal lobe, occipital lobe, and temporal lobe.

Cortical spreading depression (CSD): A pathological state in which a wave of depolarization in the cerebral cortex is followed by suppression of cerebral activity.

Cosmic radiation: Potentially harmful alpha particles, beta particles and gamma rays that originate from celestial radiation striking the earth's atmosphere.

Counseling: A type of applied psychology aimed at helping individuals challenged by emotional, behavioral, or social disorders.

Covalent bonding: A strong chemical bond formed when two atoms share electrons, resulting in the stable association of the atoms into a molecule.

CpG islands: Regions of DNA that contain a large number of cytosine-guanine repeats. The methylation status of CpG clusters has an important impact on gene expression.

CRISPR: An acronym for a gene-editing process which uses guide RNA (gRNA) bound to a CAS-9 scissors nuclease to remove dysfunctional genes and replace them with appropriate new genes. The process is enabled by DNA repair mechanisms that rapidly reconnect the DNA strands.

CSD: See *Cortical spreading depression*.

Cyclic adenosine monophosphate (cAMP): An intracellular second messenger crucial for signal transduction at the cellular level and other neurological functions. At increased concentrations, it has anti-inflammatory effects.

Cyclothymia: A relatively mild form of bipolar disorder involving brief periods of hypomania that alternate with periods of mild depression.

Cysteine: A sulfur-containing amino acid that is a constituent of many important enzymes.

Cytoplasm: The cell substance between the cell membrane and the nucleus, containing the cytosol, organelles, cytoskeleton, and various particles.

Cytosol: In neurons, a gel-like water-based substance where organelles and other cellular components reside.

d(GATC): A guanine, adenine, thymine, and cytosine (GATC) sequence that assists in mismatch repair.

Deacetylase: A class of enzymes that remove acetyl groups from histones or other molecules. Its action is opposite to that of histone acetyltransferase.

Deamination: The removal of an amino group from an amino acid or other compound.

Dendrite: The projections of a neuron specialized to receive synaptic inputs from other neurons.

Dendritic tree: A branched structure of multiple dendrites that emerge from a neuron.

Depolarization: The rapid change in membrane potential during the initial phase of a neuron firing event.

Depression: In psychology, a mental disorder characterized by persistent feelings of sadness, despair, and a loss of interest or pleasure in activities.

Diffusional forces: In biology, the natural tendency of atoms or molecules to move from an area of high concentration to an area of low concentration.

Dismutase: An antioxidant enzyme that converts superoxide free radicals to a less aggressive molecule, H_2O_2.

DNA (Deoxyribonucleic acid): A molecule that contains the genetic instructions needed for organisms to develop, grow, survive, and reproduce.

DNA adduct: A form of DNA damage involving covalent attachment of an atom or molecule to DNA.

DNA damage response (DDR): A complex network of cellular pathways that detect, signal, and repair damage to DNA strands.

DNA damage: A harmful alteration in the chemical structure of DNA, such as a break in a DNA strand, a missing nucleobase, or a foreign chemical adduct.

DNA glycosylase: A DNA repair enzyme responsible for recognizing and removing damaged or inappropriate bases from DNA.

DNA ligase: An enzyme that plays a crucial role in the repair of DNA by joining or "ligating" fragments of DNA together.

DNA methylation: A biological process in which methyl groups are added to the DNA molecule. Methylation at the C5 position of cytosine bases may reduce expression of individual genes.

DNA repair: A collection of complex processes that continuously identify and correct structural and chemical DNA damage.

Docking site: A pre-synaptic membrane site where vesicles accumulate prior to the ejection of their neurotransmitters into a synapse.

Domain: A conserved part of a given protein sequence or tertiary structure that can evolve, function, and exist independently of the rest of the protein chain.

Dopamine: A catecholamine neurotransmitter that is also a precursor of nor-epinephrine and adrenaline.

Dopamine beta-hydroxylase (DBH): A copper-containing oxygenase enzyme that converts dopamine to norepinephrine.

Dopamine receptor D2 (also known as D2R): An autoreceptor that modulates the release of dopamine and plays a role in reward and memory.

Dopamine transporter (DAT): A protein embedded in presynaptic membranes that acts as a passageway for neurotransmitters during reuptake.

Dorsal raphe (DR): A tiny brain stem nucleus in the midbrain and pons that is the major source of serotonin in the brain.

Double helix: In molecular biology, the structure formed by double-stranded molecules of nucleic acids such as DNA and RNA. The DNA double helix is a spiral polymer of nucleic acids, held together by nucleotides that base pair together.

Double-blind study: An experimental procedure in which neither the subjects of the experiment nor the persons administering the experiment know certain critical aspects of the experiment until the results have been recorded. This protocol guards against experimenter bias and enables measurement of placebo effects.

Double-strand breaks (DSBs): A form of DNA damage in which both strands of a DNA molecule are broken.

Down syndrome: A genetic disorder resulting from an extra copy of chromosome 21, causing delays, distinctive facial features, and varying levels of intellectual disability.

DSM-5-TR (Diagnostic and Statistical Manual of Mental Disorders, Fifth Edition, Text Revision): The standard classification of mental disorders used by mental health professionals, published by the American Psychiatric Association.

Dysthymia: A mild but chronic form of depression.

Electrochemistry: The branch of chemistry that deals with the relations between electrical and chemical phenomena.

Electroconvulsive therapy (ECT): Previously known as electroshock therapy; a form of treatment for major depression or mania where electrical currents are applied to a patient's skull.

Electrostatic: Relating to stationary electric charges or fields as opposed to electric currents.

End-feet: See *Astrocyte end-feet*.

Endoplasmic reticulum (ER): A network of tubular membranes within the cytoplasm of a cell, occurring either with a smooth surface (smooth endoplasmic reticulum) or studded with ribosomes (rough endoplasmic reticulum).

Entorhinal cortex: A brain region located in the medial temporal lobe that has major roles in memory, navigation, and time perception, and is the main interface between the hippocampus and the neocortex.

Entropy: A measure of disorder or randomness in a system, describing the tendency for systems to become less organized over time.

Enzyme: A protein (or conjugated protein) produced in the body that speeds up a chemical reaction.

Epigenetic disorder: A physical or psychiatric disorder caused by changes in gene expression rates.

Epigenetics: The study of changes in gene activity that do not involve alterations to the genetic code, including DNA methylation and histone modification mechanisms.

Epilepsy: A common chronic neurological disorder characterized by recurrent unprovoked seizures, caused by episodic abnormal electrical activity in the brain.

Etiology: The cause or origin of a disease or condition.

Euphoria: A feeling or state of intense excitement, happiness, and well-being.

Euthymia: In bipolar disorder, the phase between manic and depressive episodes involving a stable mood that is neither extremely elevated nor depressed.

Excitatory: In neuroscience, something that increases the likelihood of a neuron firing an action potential.

Exon: In transcription, a gene region that is attached to mRNA that assists in specifying the amino acid sequence of an expressed protein.

Extracellular: Occurring or being situated outside the cell or cells. For example, extracellular fluid is the fluid found outside the cell.

Extrapyramidal symptoms (EPS): A group of side effects that impact the motor system and are typically caused by antipsychotic medications.

Folate: A water-soluble B vitamin that occurs naturally in food, necessary for the production and maintenance of new cells, synthesis of DNA, and other functions.

Formaldehyde (CH_2O): A colorless pungent gas that can act as a long-term preservative of biological tissues.

Free radical: An atom or molecule that has an unpaired electron in its outer shell that can react with and damage biological structures.

Functional magnetic resonance imaging (fMRI): A noninvasive procedure that measures brain activity by detecting chances in blood flow.

GABA (γ-Aminobutyric acid): The chief inhibitory neurotransmitter in the central nervous system.

Gap junction: A specialized connection between cells that allows the passage of molecules, ions, or electrical impulses.

GATC sequence: The sequence of DNA's four nucleotides (guanine, adenine, thymine, and cytosine) in specific DNA sites and proteins.

Gene: A hereditary unit consisting of a sequence of DNA that occupies a specific location on a chromosome and determines a particular characteristic in an organism.

Gene expression: The process by which information from a gene is used in the synthesis of a protein.

Genetic concordance: The presence of the same trait or characteristic in both members of a pair of twins.

Genetics: The branch of biology that deals with heredity, especially the mechanisms of hereditary transmission and the variation of inherited characteristics among similar or related organisms.

Genome: The entirety of an organism's hereditary information, including both the genes and the non-coding sequences of its DNA.

Genome-wide association study (GWAS): An international collaborative search for DNA variants that are associated with a trait or disorder.

Gestation: The period during which a baby develops inside the mother's body before birth.

Glial cells: In the brain, non-neuronal cells that provide physical support and nutrition for neurons. In addition, they play a crucial role in brain development and neurotransmission.

Global DNA methylation: The overall methyl content of a person's DNA across their entire genome. The presence or absence of methylated cytosine at a gene's promoter region regulates its rate of gene expression.

Glutamate: The most abundant neurotransmitter in the brain. Activity at glutamate receptors is excitatory (promotes neuron firing).

Glutamine: The most abundant free amino acid in blood and a precursor of glutamate.

Glutathione (GSH): An important antioxidant found naturally in the body. It is a tripeptide composed of three amino acids (glycine, cysteine, and glutamic acid).

Glutathione peroxidase: An enzyme that protects against oxidative damage, primarily by catalyzing the reaction between glutathione (GSH) and hydrogen peroxide (H_2O_2).

Glycogen synthase kinase-3 beta (GSK-3β): A protein that helps regulate immune responses and is associated with cell death and proliferation.

Glycosylase: A molecule that starts the process of DNA base excision repair by removing the base from the helix's "backbone."

Goldman equation: Determines the net voltage (potential) across a membrane that experiences concentration gradients from more than a single ion channel type.

Golgi apparatus: An organelle (or structure) found around the nucleus of a cell that processes proteins and fats produced in the reticulum and prepares them for export outside the nucleus.

G-protein-coupled receptor (GPCR): Receptor that does not directly open a pore but sends a second messenger or other stimulus to open a pore at a different membrane site.

Graded potential: In neuroscience, a temporary voltage change in a neuron membrane that fails to reach threshold voltage and gradually fades away.

Granulocytosis: A condition wherein granulocytes, a type of white blood cell, increase in peripheral blood. This condition is a symptom of several illnesses.

GSH: See *Glutathione.*

GSK-3β: See *Glycogen synthase kinase-3 beta.*

Guanine: One of the four constituent bases of DNA.

Guillain-Barre syndrome (GBS): A condition in which the immune system attacks the nerves.

GWAS: See *Genome-wide association study.*

Hayflick limit: The number of times a normal cell can divide (typically 40–60 times) before it fails to function effectively.

Hippocampus: A region of the brain's temporal lobe that plays an important role in learning and memory.

Histamine: A naturally occurring organic compound that is a brain neurotransmitter and also has a major role in allergic reactions, immunity, and inflammation.

Histone: Linear alkaline proteins that develop a ball-type configuration and provide structural support for DNA that winds around it. They are major protein components of chromatin and play a role in gene regulation.

Histone modification: Epigenetic alteration of gene expression due to specific chemical reactions at histone tails.

Histone tail: Linear histone segments that protrude from nucleosomes that have an important role in regulating gene expression or silencing.

Hormone: In biology, a chemical produced by an endocrine gland that travels to target cells and tissues, influencing their activity and functions.

Hydrolase: An enzyme that uses water to break chemical bonds, typically dividing larger molecules into smaller ones.

Hydroxide ion (OH^-): A negatively charged ion formed when a water molecule loses a hydrogen ion (H^+).

Hyperactivity: A physical state in which a person is easily excitable or exuberant, often resulting in strong emotional reactions, impulsive behavior, and a short attention span. In brain neurons, the condition of increased firing rates.

Hypermethylation: In DNA, a condition in which excessive methyl groups (CH_3) attach to DNA, often leading to gene silencing. In biochemistry, elevated activity of methylase enzymes.

Hypersexuality: A condition in which a person experiences overly increased sexual desires and compulsions that may cause impairments in quality of life.

Hypoactivity: A medical condition involving reduced or decreased activity. In brain neurons, a condition of slowed firing rates.

Hypomania: A mild form of mania associated with Bipolar 2 disorder.

Immune function: A complex network of tissues, organs, cells, and chemicals that protects the body from infection and illness.

Impulsivity: A type of behavior characterized by a tendency to act without prior reflection or thought.

In utero: The period during which a fetus develops inside the mother's uterus (womb).

In vivo neuroimaging: The process of non-invasively studying the structure and function of the brain while the subject is still alive.

Inactivation gate: A molecular complex that stabilizes closed ion channels and prevents reopening.

Inflammation: A localized protective reaction of tissue to irritation, injury, or infection, characterized by pain, redness, swelling, and sometimes loss of function.

Intron: A non-coding sequence within a gene that is removed during RNA splicing in translation.

Ion: An atom or molecule with a net electric charge resulting from the gain or loss of one or more electrons.

Ion channel: Protein structures that snake in and out of neuronal membranes and provide passageways for ions.

Ion channel pump: A transmembrane protein that moves ions across a plasma membrane against their concentration gradient.

Ionizing radiation: High-energy radiation that has the potential to remove tightly bound electrons from atoms, leading to ionization and potentially causing damage to biological tissues.

Isoform: Any of two functionally similar proteins that have a similar but not identical amino acid sequence.

JNK: See *c-Jun N-terminal kinase*.

Kindling: In neurology, a theory that a seizure or other brain event can incrementally and permanently increase risk for the event to happen again.

Knockout studies: An experimental study in which a single gene is deleted from an animal or organism in order to study the effect of its absence.

Ku (Ku70/Ku80): A DNA-binding protein involved in DNA repair.

Leak channel: A membrane ion channel that is always open.

Ligase IV (LIG4): A protein that repairs double-strand DNA breaks using the non-homologous end-joining pathway.

lincRNA: See *Long intergenic non-coding RNA*.

Lithium (Li): A chemical element with atomic number 3 that is readily ionized. In biology, lithium compounds are commonly used in treatment of bipolar disorder and other mental conditions.

Loaded mRNA: In neuroscience, an mRNA molecule that has completed the coding of a protein during the translation process.

Lobotomy: A discredited, out-of-date surgical procedure where the connections of the prefrontal cortex are severed.

Locus coeruleus (LC): A small group of neurons in the brainstem that is the primary source of the neurotransmitter norepinephrine (noradrenaline).

Long intergenic non-coding RNA (lincRNA): Integral components of signaling pathways in various cancer genes.

Lymph: A colorless fluid containing white blood cells which bathes our cells.

Lymphopenia: Also known as lymphocytopenia, a condition involving abnormally low levels of white blood cells that protect against infection.

Lysosome: Cell organelle involved in digestion and waste removal.

M current: An outward-flowing K^+ current through a specific voltage-gated K^+ channel in neurons.

Magnetic resonance imaging (MRI): A medical or research technique that uses a strong magnetic field and radio waves to produce detailed images of the body's internal structures.

Magnetic resonance spectroscopy (MRS): A non-invasive technique that uses MRI scanners to examine brain metabolism by analyzing biochemical signals.

Major depression disorder (MDD): A severe type of clinical depression characterized by persistent low mood, loss of interest or pleasure, and other symptoms that interfere with daily functioning.

Mania: A state of abnormally elevated mood, energy, and activity that lasts for at least one week.

Manic depression: An obsolete term for bipolar depression.

MAO inhibitor: An antidepressant medication that elevates serotonin activity by blocking monoamine oxidase, an enzyme that metabolizes (destroys) serotonin.

Mass-transport: A scientific discipline involving diffusive and convective transport of chemical species within a physical system.

Mendelian genetics: The laws of inheritance relating to the transmission of hereditary characteristics from parents to their offspring.

Meninges: Three layers of protective membranes (dura matter, pia matter, and arachnoid matter) that stabilize the brain and spinal cord.

Messenger RNA (mRNA): A type of RNA that copies a gene's code and delivers it to ribosomes for the production of a specific protein.

Metal metabolism: In biochemistry, metabolic processes aimed at providing appropriate concentrations of metal ions for enzymatic and other chemical reactions.

Metalloenzyme: Proteins that contain metal ions that are involved in chemical reactions.

Metallothionein: A family of four low molecular weight cysteine-rich proteins that have potent metal binding and redox capabilities and are involved in early brain development. They have powerful antioxidant properties and work together with glutathione and selenium to protect against toxic metals.

Methyl group: A reactive chemical entity with formula CH_3 that participates in many dozens of biochemical reactions.

Methyl mark (abbreviation for methyl bookmark): A stable epigenetic positioning of a methyl group on DNA gene sites that regulates the gene's expression rate.

Methylation: The addition of a methyl group to a molecule or atom; a primary factor in epigenetic modification of gene expression.

Methylenetetrahydrofolate reductase (MTHFR): An enzyme that plays a crucial role in the metabolism of folate (vitamin B9).

Methyltransferase: An enzyme that transfers a methyl group to a molecule, often playing a role in DNA regulation and gene expression.

MGMT (O6-methylguanine methyltransferase): A repair enzyme that directly removes methyl group adducts from guanine nucleotides in DNA.

Microglia: Tiny glial cells surrounding brain neurons that provide immunity, repair damaged neurons, and remove brain waste.

Micron: A unit of distance equal to one-millionth of a meter.

MicroRNA (miRNA): Small, non-coding RNA molecules that primarily function in transcriptional regulation of gene expression, including the elimination of improper mRNA transcripts.

Microtubules: Rod-shaped components of brain neurons that provide structural support for the axon, serve as a conduit for nutrients and organelles, and participate in cellular processes including mitosis. They are generally straight and about 24 nanometers in diameter.

Millimoles per liter (mM). A concentration unit equal to one-thousandth of a mole per liter.

Millivolt (mV): One-thousandth of a volt.

Mismatch repair (MMR): A repair process that corrects errors in DNA replication in which an improper base is present in the DNA strand.

Missense: In genetics, a mutation in a codon that results in production of an improper amino acid.

Mitochondria: A double-membrane organelle in the cytoplasm of cells that supplies energy and enables cell respiration.

Mitosis: A type of cell division that results in two daughter cells each having the same number and kind of chromosomes as the parent nucleus.

MMR: See *Mismatch repair.*

Molecular biology: The study of biology at a molecular level, including the molecular nature of DNA, RNA and the mechanisms of gene replication, mutation, and expression. This field combines the sciences of biology and chemistry and studies the mechanisms and kinetics of cellular and tissue processes.

Monoamine oxidase (MAO): A family of enzymes that oxidize (break down) neurotransmitters at the synapse, reducing the population of those neurotransmitters and lowering synaptic activity.

MRE11: A double-strand repair protein encoded by the *MRE11* gene.

MRI: See *Magnetic resonance imaging.*

MRN complex: A protein network involved in sensing, processing, and repairing double-strand breaks.

mRNA: See *Messenger RNA.*

MRS: See *Magnetic resonance spectroscopy.*

MTHFR: See *Methylenetetrahydrofolate reductase.*

Multiple sclerosis (MS): A chronic, typically progressive disease involving damage to the myelin coverings of nerve cells in the brain and spinal cord.

Mutation: A change in the DNA sequence of an organism which may be inborn or result from errors during DNA replication, exposure to mutagens, or other factors.

MutH: An endonuclease enzyme involved in DNA mismatch repair.

Myelin: A structure of lipid fats and proteins that forms a sheath around the axons of neurons. Myelin provides electrical insulation and physical support for the cell and facilitates the transmission of nerve signals along the axon.

Myo-inositol: The most common form of inositol, a sugar alcohol that helps the body process insulin.

N-acetylcysteine (NAC): An important antioxidant in all humans that protects against oxidative stress. It is a popular supplement available in pharmacies and health food stores.

N-acetylaspartate (NAA): The acetylated form of the amino acid aspartate that is present exclusively in the nervous system.

N-glycosidic bond: A type of chemical bond that connects a nitrogenous base to the sugar component of a nucleotide in DNA or RNA.

N-methyl-D-aspartate receptor (NMDAR) : A complex type of glutamate receptor that requires simultaneous activation by glutamate and an amino acid such as D-serine or glycine. These glutamate receptors have a major role in learning and memory and abnormal functioning is associated with schizophrenia and other mental disorders.

Natural killer cells (NK cells): A type of immune cell that can kill tumor cells or cells infected with a virus.

Nernst equation: A mathematical formula that determines the potential (voltage) across a cell membrane containing a single type of ion channel.

Neurobiology: Commonly referred to as neuroscience, the study of molecular, developmental, structural, functional, and medical aspects of the nervous system.

Neurochemistry: The study of neurotransmitters, psychiatric drugs, and other molecules that influence brain function.

Neurodegeneration: The progressive loss of structure or function of brain cells, usually culminating in the death of the cells.

Neuron: An electrically excitable nerve cell that processes and transmits information to other neurons by electrical and chemical signaling across a synapse. Neurons interact with each other to form networks and are the core components of the brain and peripheral nervous system.

Neuron firing: An expression that refers to an action potential resulting in the release of neurotransmitters into a synapse.

Neuronal hyperactivity: Abnormally elevated rate of neuronal action potentials (neuron firing events).

Neuronal pruning: The process by which excess neurons and synaptic connections are eliminated in order to increase the efficiency of neuronal transmissions. Also called 'synaptic pruning,' this process is especially active during early development and after puberty onset.

Neuroscience: A science dealing with the structure or function of the nervous system and brain.

Neurotransmission: The process in which signals are transmitted between nerve cells (neurons) in the brain and nervous system.

Neurotransmitter: A chemical that is released from a neuron and transmits an impulse to another neuron. A neurotransmitter is a messenger of information from one neuron to another. Many dozens of neurotransmitters have been identified, including monoamines, amino acids, peptides, and other chemicals such as acetylcholine, zinc, and nitric oxide.

Nodes of Ranvier: Regularly spaced gaps in an axon's myelin sheath that contain voltage-gated Na^+ ion channels that provide a power boost during action potentials.

Non-coding RNA: A functional RNA molecule that doesn't code for a protein.

Norepinephrine (NE): A catecholamine neurotransmitter synthesized from dopamine that also functions as a stress hormone. Elevated levels have been associated with anxiety and panic disorders, with depressed levels associated with catatonic tendencies.

Nucleosome: The basic unit of DNA packaging, consisting of a segment of DNA wound around a histone protein core.

Nucleotide: One of several organic molecules that are building blocks of DNA and RNA, consisting of a ribose or deoxyribose sugar joined to a purine or pyrimidine base and to a phosphate group.

Nutrient: A nourishing food substance that provides energy or is necessary for growth and repair. Examples of nutrients are vitamins, minerals, carbohydrates, fats, and proteins.

Obsessive-compulsive disorder (OCD): A mental and behavioral disorder characterized by uncontrollable recurring thoughts, repetitive actions, and high anxiety.

Off-target: Unwanted changes in non-targeted DNA genes caused by CRISPR or other gene-editing approaches aimed at replacing non-functional genes.

OGG1: See *8-oxoguanine DNA glycosylase*.

Oligodendrocyte: A type of glial cell that forms myelin sheaths that insulate neuronal axons.

One-carbon cycle: In biology, a chemical cycle in which (a) dietary protein (methionine) is converted to a molecule (SAMe) that readily donates methyl groups for various reactions in the body, and (b) methionine levels are conserved by a series of chemical reactions.

$ONOO^-$ (peroxynitrite): A highly reactive, damaging free radical formed from the reaction of superoxide and nitric oxide.

Organelle: A membrane-enclosed structure inside a cell. Examples include the nucleus, Golgi apparatus, and mitochondria.

Oxidation: A process where a substance loses electrons, gains oxygen, or loses hydrogen.

Oxidative overload: A condition in which the body has too many free radicals and not enough antioxidants to combat their harmful effects.

p53 gene: A tumor suppressor gene located on chromosome 17.

p53 network: An intricate system of genes and proteins regulated by the tumor suppressor gene *p53*.

p53 protein: A DNA repair protein expressed by the *p53* gene.

PANDAS (pediatric autoimmune neuropsychiatric disorder): A medical condition associated with streptococcal infections.

Paranoia: A psychological disorder characterized by delusions of persecution or grandeur.

Parkinson's disease: A progressive disorder of the central nervous system associated with the degeneration of dopamine neurons in the substantia nigra area of the brain. Common symptoms are high-frequency tremors, muscle rigidity, slowed physical movements, an abnormal gait, impaired speech, and loss of facial expressions.

PARP1: An enzyme that assists in DNA repair, chromatin remodeling, and gene repair.

Pathology: The study of the essential nature of diseases, especially of the structural and functional changes produced by them.

Peptide: Any compound composed of a series of amino acids linked by covalent bonds.

Permeability: In neurons, the relative ease with which an ion can cross the bilayer membrane through an open leak channel.

Peroxynitrite: See *ONOO⁻*.

Phosphate: Any of various salts or esters of phosphoric acid, characterized by a PO_4 chemical group.

Phosphorylation: The addition of a phosphate group to a molecule, typically a protein, which can regulate its activity or function.

Pia mater: One of three protective membranes that cover the brain. It clings tightly to the exterior of the brain and is distinguished by delicate connective tissue with many tiny blood vessels.

Placebo effect: Improvement in the condition of an experimental subject that is not related to the treatment under study. The improvements may be due either to psychological expectations of benefits or changes in the environment unknown to the experimenter.

Plasma: The fluid part of blood.

Plasticity: In neuroscience, the ability of an organism to change its physical, behavioral, or physiological traits in response to environmental conditions.

Polarity: In biology, the differences that exist in electrical charge or other factors between opposite sides of a molecule, cell, or organism.

Polypharmacy: The simultaneous use of multiple drugs by a patient.

Pore: In neuroscience, a minute opening in a structure through which ions or other biochemical entities can pass.

Post-traumatic stress disorder (PTSD): A mental and behavioral disorder that develops from experiencing a traumatic event, such as military combat, violent assaults, or other threats to a person's life or wellbeing.

Postpartum depressive disorder (PPD): Also known as postnatal depression, a form of clinical depression that develops after having a baby. This disorder typically involves extreme anxiety, frequent crying, fatigue, and hopelessness. Severe cases may involve psychosis and suicidal ideation.

Potassium (K): A chemical element with atomic number 19. A soft silvery-white reactive metal of the alkali metal group.

Potential (also known as voltage): In neuroscience, the imbalance of electrical charge between the interior of electrically excitable neurons and their surroundings.

Prader-Willi syndrome (PWS): A genetic disorder that causes intellectual disability, obesity, and shortness in height.

Predisposition: In biology, a tendency to acquire a condition or quality, usually based on the combined effects of genetic and environmental factors.

Prefrontal cortex (PFC): A region of the brain located in the frontal lobe that enables higher-order cognitive capabilities, including planning, decision-making, working memory, and other executive functions.

Presynaptic membrane proteins: Specialized proteins in the vesicle wall, presynaptic membrane, and cytosol that assist vesicle docking, formation of a fusion pore, sensing of Ca^{++}, and neurotransmitter release.

Presynaptic membrane: The part of an axon terminal's membrane that faces adjacent brain cells across a synapse gap and emits neurotransmitters that may activate the adjacent cell.

Progenitor cells: Early descendants of stem cells that can differentiate to form one or more cell types but cannot divide and reproduce indefinitely.

Promoter region: Regions of DNA located upstream of a gene, providing a control point for regulation of gene expression.

Protein: A molecule composed of amino acids in a specific sequence determined by the DNA coding for the protein. Proteins are required for the structure, function, and regulation of the body's cells, tissues, and organs.

Protoplasm: A colorless, jelly-like substance that makes up the living parts of plant and animal cells.

Psychodynamic therapy: A form of treatment that explores the unconscious mind and its influence on current thoughts, feelings, and behaviors.

Psychomotor retardation (PR): A slowing of mental and physical abilities.

Psychosis: A symptom or feature of mental illness usually characterized by radical changes in personality, impaired functioning, and a distorted sense of objective reality (hallucinations, delusions, paranoia, etc.).

Psychotherapy: Also called talk therapy, a process whereby psychological problems are treated through communication and relationship factors between an individual and a trained mental health professional.

Psychotropic medication: A drug that can treat symptoms related to mood, behavior, perception, or thoughts.

Pyrimidine base: A nitrogenous base found in nucleic acids (DNA and RNA).

Pyrrole: Any of a class of organic compounds of the heterocyclic series with a ring structure of four carbon atoms and one nitrogen atom. Specific pyrrole molecules have biological properties that may have harmful or therapeutic impacts on a person.

Radial glia: Bipolar-shaped progenitor cells that are responsible for producing neurons, astrocytes, oligodendrocytes, and microglia in the brain.

Raphe nuclei: A moderate-size cluster of neurons found in the brainstem that produce serotonin and release this neurotransmitter to the rest of the brain.

Reactive nitrogen species (RNS): A group of chemically reactive molecules including ONOO⁻ that can cause severe DNA damage. RNS molecules perform important biochemical functions at normal concentrations but are harmful at higher levels.

Reactive oxidative species (ROS): A class of highly reactive molecules that contain oxygen and may cause severe damage to DNA, RNA, proteins, and cells.

Receptor: In neuroscience, a protein embedded in a neuronal membrane that interacts with neurotransmitters to enhance or inhibit action potentials (neuron firing).

Rectify: In neuroscience, a process of correcting or making something right.

Refractory period: A brief period after depolarization during which a neuron cannot fire again.

Repolarization: In neuroscience, a neuron's return to resting voltage after an action potential.

Resting potential: The steady-state voltage of a neuron when it is not generating an action potential.

Reticulum: In the context of brain neurons, a network of membrane-bound sacs and tubules that have crucial roles in protein synthesis, lipid metabolism, and calcium regulation.

Reuptake: A process by which a neurotransmitter in a synapse is returned to the original brain cell, usually facilitated by a special transmembrane transporter protein.

ROS: See *Reactive oxygen species*.

Rough endoplasmic reticulum (RER): A cell organelle that assists in protein production, folding, and calcium storage.

SAMe (S-adenosyl-L-methionine): A molecule produced by an enzymatic reaction between methionine and ATP (adenosine triphosphate). SAMe is the primary methyl donor for 80+ methylase reactions in the body and is regulated by the one-carbon cycle.

Schizophrenia: Any of several psychotic disorders that commonly involve auditory hallucinations, paranoid or bizarre delusions, disorganized speech, anxiety, depression, and other symptoms that usually result in significant social and occupational deficits.

Second messengers: In neurotransmission, small molecules and ions that relay signals from activated post-synaptic receptors to other membrane areas to open a pore.

Selective serotonin reuptake inhibitors (SSRIs): A family of antidepressant medications that increase serotonin activity by inhibiting reuptake of serotonin from synapses.

Senescence: In biology, a process by which a cell ages and stops dividing but does not die.

Serotonin (5-hydroxytryptamine or 5-HT): In brain, a monoamine neurotransmitter biochemically derived from tryptophan that has an important role in depression and other mental disorders.

Serotonin transporter (SERT): A specialized protein that terminates serotonin signaling by using sodium and chloride gradients to drive reuptake of serotonin into presynaptic membranes.

Serotonin-norepinephrine reuptake inhibitor (SNRI): An antidepressant medication that increases the levels of serotonin and norepinephrine in the brain.

Serum: In blood, the clear yellowish fluid liquid that remains after fibrinogen and other clotting factions have been removed from plasma.

Side effect: In medicine, a secondary effect of a drug or other treatment that may be undesirable.

Signaling: Often referred to as signal transduction or transmembrane signaling, the process by which cells or other biochemical entities sense external cues from their external environment.

Single nucleotide polymorphism (SNP): In genetics, a variant of a DNA's amino acid sequence that may alter the structure or function of an expressed protein.

Single-strand break: A form of DNA damage in which one strand of the DNA duplex is severed.

Smooth endoplasmic reticulum (SER): In neurons, a large and complex tubular network that stores and regulates calcium levels, assists axonal repair, neurite growth, and neurotransmissions.

SOD1 (also called Cu Zn SOD1): A dismutase enzyme that rectifies superoxide free radicals in neuronal cytosol.

SOD2 (also called Mn SOD2): A dismutase enzyme that rectifies superoxide free radicals formed in the mitochondria.

SOD3 (also called Cu Zn SOD3): A dismutase enzyme that rectifies superoxide free radicals outside neuronal membranes.

Sodium-potassium pump: An enzyme also known as the Na^+/K^+ pump or Na^+/K^+-ATPase found in cell membranes that exports sodium ions and imports potassium ions to form an electric potential (voltage).

Sodium (Na): Chemical element with atomic number 11, a soft silver-white reactive metal of the alkali metal group.

Soma: The largest part of a neuron that contains the nucleus and other essential organelles, serving as the neuro's metabolic and informational center.

Spatial buffering: In neuroscience, a mechanism that assists the removal of extracellular potassium by astrocytes.

Spatial summation: A neural process where multiple incoming inputs from different dendrites are combined to determine the proximity to the threshold voltage.

Spreading depression (SD): Refers to severely depressed neuronal activity that can quickly (and briefly) spread across neural tissues.

Staging model: In psychology, a theoretical framework that divides a process into consecutive distinct stages, each characterized by qualitatively different mechanisms and functions.

Steady state: A condition in which a system is stable and balanced with equal rates of inputs and outputs, resulting in no overall change in the system over a specific time.

Substantia nigra: A brain structure in the basal ganglia that is the primary site for dopamine synthesis and activity.

Subventricular zone (SVZ): A term used to describe both embryonic and adult neural tissues in the brain. During the nine months of gestation, the SVZ refers to a secondary proliferative zone containing neural progenitor cells which divide to produce new neurons.

SUMOylation: A post-translational modification in which a small ubiquitin-like modifier (SUMO) protein attaches to cells experiencing DNA damage and influences the risk of senescence, apoptosis, cancer, or continuing cell function.

Superoxide dismutase (SOD): A family of three metalloenzymes that provide important antioxidant protection by converting superoxide free radicals to less aggressive hydrogen peroxide and oxygen.

Suprachiasmatic nuclei (SCN): A small part of the brain's hypothalamus that regulates the timing of sleep, wakefulness, body temperature, and hormone secretion.

Synapse: The space between neurons that allows them to communicate by passing neurotransmitter signals.

Synthesis: The production of a substance by the union of chemical elements, groups, or simpler compounds, or by the degradation of a complex compound.

Tardive dyskinesia: Potential side-effects of antipsychotic medications that may include uncontrollable stiff, jerky movements.

Temporal summation: Multiple rapidly occurring stimuli occurring at a single synapse location.

Thiol redox: Oxidation-reduction reactions involving thiol compounds that contain a sulfhydryl group (-SH).

Threshold voltage: In neurons, the critical level to which a membrane potential must be depolarized to initiate an action potential.

Tight junctions: In brain, transmembrane protein complexes that line the interior of blood vessels to form a semi-impermeable barrier that prevents passage of large molecules, toxins, and pathogens, while allowing passage of small molecules and gases.

Tissue-staining: Application of colored dyes or other substances that highlight and improve the contrast of microscopic tissue components.

Transcription factor (TF): In molecular biology, a protein that affects the rate of transcription of genetic information from DNA to messenger RNA.

Transcription: In biology, the first step in gene expression in which its specific amino acid sequence is copied onto a mRNA molecule.

Translation: In biology, a process in which proteins are produced at cell ribosomes using mRNA molecules as templates.

Transmembrane protein: A protein that spans the entire cell membrane and acts as a conduit for nutrients, neurotransmitters, or other substances that may enter or leave the cell.

Transporter protein: In neurotransmission, a membrane-spanning protein which enables rapid reuptake of a neurotransmitter from the synapse.

Trauma: A physical or emotional response to a deeply distressing or disturbing event.

Treatment-emergent affective switch (TEAS): The emergence of a manic or hypomanic episode in a person with bipolar disorder after starting or changing a medication or other treatment.

Tricyclic antidepressant: A class of antidepressant medications characterized by a three-ring chemical structure, with side chains containing a tertiary amine.

Triple-helix model: Linus Pauling's disproved model of DNA structure with three intertwined strands instead of the now-accepted double helix.

Tryptophan: An essential amino acid needed for the synthesis of serotonin, growth in infancy, and nitrogen balance in adults.

Twin studies: Research investigations which examine differences or similarities between identical and fraternal twins.

Ubiquitin: A small protein comprised of 76 amino acids that is present in all human cells and plays a role in cell signaling, senescence, apoptosis (cell death), DNA repair and other functions.

Undermethylation: A below-normal content of methyl groups in DNA that may increase expression of many genes. Alternatively, a weakness in the 80+ methylase enzymes in the body's periphery.

Uric acid: A nitrogen-containing compound that is a byproduct of purine metabolism in the body.

UvrABC endonuclease (NER): A bacterial multienzyme complex involved in nucleotide excision repair.

Vedas: A collection of hymns and other ancient religious texts written in India between 1500 and 1000 B.C.

Vesicles: Tiny bubble-like membrane-enclosed structures in brain neurons that store and transport neurotransmitters and other cellular products.

Vitamin: Any of various fat-soluble or water-soluble organic substances essential in minute amounts for normal growth and activity of the body and obtained naturally from plant and animal foods.

VMAT (vesicular monoamine transporter): A transport protein embedded in the membrane of a vesicle that facilitates the loading of neurotransmitter molecules into a vesicle.

Voltage-gated ion channels (VGICs): Transmembrane proteins that are normally closed but allow passage of ions when membrane voltage reaches a specific threshold potential.

Writing, Reading, and Erasing: The major epigenetic approaches for adjusting expression of a specific gene.

X-ray crystallography: A scientific technique that employs X-rays to determine the detailed structure of molecules, aiding in understanding atomic arrangements within the molecule.

XLF: A protein crucial for non-homologous end joining, a primary pathway for repairing double strand DNA breaks.

Zinc depletion: A medical condition involving insufficient amounts of the mineral zinc for the body's essential functions.

Zinc fingers: A family of small zinc metalloproteins that have a role in genetic transcription and other processes, typically acting as interaction modules that bind to DNA, RNA, proteins, or small molecules.

The following pages are provided for notes.